John Plimmer

THE WHITECHAPEL MURDERS – SOLVED?

An Examination of the Jack the Ripper Murders
Using Modern Police Techniques

HOUSE OF STRATUS

This edition published in 2003 by House of Stratus, an imprint of House of Stratus Ltd, Thirsk Industrial Park, York Road, Thirsk, North Yorkshire, YO7 3BX, UK.

www.houseofstratus.com

Typeset by House of Stratus, printed and bound by Short Run Press Limited.

A catalogue record for this book is available from the British Library and the Library of Congress.

ISBN 0-7551-1365-9

Contents

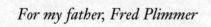

For my father, Fred Plimmer

Introduction

Victorian Whitechapel was very different from the buildings and highways that exist today. Dark and poorly lit cobbled streets with dingy terraced properties surrounded by poverty were all too common in many areas of nineteenth-century Britain. The East End of London was no exception. Rolling mists and burning gas lamps would frequently meet the dusk. The darkness of night would encourage prostitutes, rogues and vagabonds onto the streets. The majority of the working population sought refuge in tiny back-street public houses and other seedy places of entertainment, providing escapism from the daily trauma and misery associated with the lower classes residing in the area.

'Inner-city Victorians' possessed characteristics that have not been so prevalent in recent years. Crimes of child neglect, domestic violence and cruelty were regarded with insensitivity and acceptance. Prostitution was commonplace, although not spoken of as freely and openly as it is today. Illiteracy was infectious, and lower-class women had to focus more on survival rather than education. There wasn't much middle ground amongst people, and extreme views and reactions to situations existed more so than today. Daily episodes that varied from the usual and accepted way of life were dealt with by excitement or silence, tears or laughter, happiness or depression. Pockets of turmoil and confusion still existed as a result of the unemployment riots of 1886 and 1887, and destitution had increased to a level where it was becoming recognized as a normal way of life. There was undoubtedly a fast-growing need for social reform.

During the summer of 1888, the people of Whitechapel had no idea of the black clouds about to descend upon them. The great London dock strike was about to take place in the following year, but only after other events had introduced fear, distress and disruption to the local neighbourhoods – a series of murders that would be the subject of investigation and debate for the next one hundred years or more.

What took place during that autumn left a nation shocked and devastated and was responsible for one of the most talked about mysteries ever recorded in British criminal history. The search for a brutal and sadistic killer, wanted for a number of terrifying murders, was never to be resolved conclusively. Five horrific slayings of human beings that would remain on Scotland Yard's books as undetected. The residents of Whitechapel were subjected to all the upheaval and trepidation associated with the butchering of five common prostitutes living and working within their own community. Both horror and panic spread like an uncontrollable disease throughout the country's capital, so much so that at one stage there was concern that anarchy would prevail over law and order. The very foundations of Victorian society were shaken with such effect that there has never since been a repeat of the consequences, which almost brought about the downfall of a government. The person responsible was never caught and may have continued to stalk the streets of London until his natural death. He was known as 'Jack the Ripper'.

The following chapters tell the story of each murder. Details have been taken from records made at the time and from a number of observations made by previous authors, criminologists and researchers. Policing methods have progressed considerably since the turn of the last century. The methods used by detective officers to tackle prolonged major investigations are explained in detail. The principal objective of this book is to outline the techniques and procedures used today. The structuring of Major Incident Rooms and the strategic and operational planning that drives a murder inquiry are described fully. The aim is not to solve the Whitechapel murders or to establish the probable identity of Jack the Ripper, but to compare the levels of professionalism and methods used in 1888 with current practices and procedures, and to identify some of those facilities that were not available a hundred years ago.

Even today, the Forensic Science Service is working towards linking genetic profiling with facial characteristics. For example, one particular gene found in blood or other samples taken from the scene of a crime could identify a person's ancestry or race. Another gene could disclose the fact that an individual's hair is red in colour. Other facial characteristics, such as the size of a nose or ears, could be valuable information towards obtaining an accurate description of a criminal. Once specific facial features have been recognized, categories could be created into which suspects would be placed. The current research is aimed towards assisting the investigating police officer in identifying offenders. There is a great deal of optimism that future development of DNA profiling could dramatically increase the success rate of linking suspects with crime scenes.

Perhaps historically the Ripper murders were not the most difficult to investigate, but they were certainly the most violent and emotive. Since the crimes were committed, there has been a great deal of focused analysis and research study completed on them. The circumstances of the murders have been well documented. The following chapters contain brief descriptions of background information to each of the incidents. Comparisons are then made with current investigative methods, as if the Victorian police officers had access to twenty-first-century facilities. References are made to Genetic Fingerprinting, Crime Pattern Analysis, the use of information technology in major investigations, and other present and accepted methods.

The question as to whether or not Jack the Ripper would have been caught if he had committed the murders during the late twentieth century, must obviously remain unanswered. However the investigations that were completed in 1888 are transported forward to the present time, together with the principal clues extracted from each of the Ripper's crimes. They are analysed and dealt with in the policing environment that exists today: the investigative arena of the twenty-first century. It is then for the reader to decide whether or not the Ripper would have been brought to justice one hundred years on.

The facts extracted from the Victorian murders are meshed into the strategic planning and structuring methods adopted by senior investigating officers who deal with current murder cases. Some fiction has been introduced to simplify the inter-pretation of procedures and practices adopted in 1888, and to compare those historical methods with current policies and routine procedures. The developments and variations which have been created by the passage of time are identified and discussed.

The second part of the book is aimed towards concluding current methods of investigation. A fictitious story has been developed, to enable the reader to assess a likely outcome to a similar series of murders that have taken place 'one hundred years on'. The procedures and techniques referred to are, however, factual and widely practised throughout the police service today.

The tensions and stress experienced by senior investigating officers, commonly associated with the management of high-profile investigations, are also described and examined.

Comparisons are made between the pressures that would have existed in the Ripper enquiries and those which current senior investigators have to deal with. It is suggested that those ordeals which result from failure to detect high-profile crimes in a short period of time are no different from those that existed in 1888.

In recent years criminal investigation has progressed in leaps and bounds, particularly in the fields of forensic science and information technology. The reader will be able to share in the operational planning of a twentieth-century senior investigating officer given the task of identifying the serial killer known as 'Jack the Ripper'.

One

Mary Ann Nichols

'The killing of a human being by a human being'

Mary Ann, 'Polly' Nichols lived in a doss-house at 18 Thrawl Street, Spitalfields, for several weeks prior to her murder. It was a dirty and smelly abode, typical of many such residences that existed throughout London during the late Victorian period. She paid up to fourpence a night for her bed and drink, out of the coppers she earned from prostitution. Although a married woman, Mary had not seen her husband William Nichols for three years. Their time together had been a tumultuous one involving drunken brawls, which had usually resulted in the husband being seriously assaulted.

For a short while she went to live with her father, who was a blacksmith in Camberwell. More drunken quarrels took place, and Mary eventually left to enter the employment of a family named Cowdry who resided in Rose Hill Road, Wandsworth. There she remained until 12 July 1888, when it was alleged that she was dismissed for theft. The weeks that followed were spent either at the Thrawl Street address or in other common lodging-houses.

There were five children from Mary's marriage to William Nichols, but they all resided with relatives or in local care homes. On the day before her untimely death she had been evicted from the squalor where she lived because of a lack of funds to pay for the rent. However on the night of Thursday, 30 August 1888, her luck changed. Mary Nichols earned sufficient pennies for a bed for the night from two clients. Full of gin, tired and heavy-eyed, she staggered through the damp and foggy backstreets looking for a night's sleep.

George Cross, a market worker in nearby Spitalfields, was still a little groggy after only a few hours' sleep, as he walked towards his place of employment. It was 3.45 a.m. on Friday, 31 August 1888. Head bowed and with hands in pockets, he listened to the echoes of his own footsteps as he walked into Bucks Row, hardly noticing the dingy smell that drifted upwards from the gutters as a reminder to passers-by of the dirt and poverty existing in that part of London. When reaching a point opposite a slaughterhouse known as Barbers, situated halfway down the street, Cross glanced up and saw what appeared to be an untidy pile of clothing on the pavement opposite. At first he thought it could be something of benefit for himself, and looked around to ensure no one else was about. He scurried across the street towards the bundle, but stopped. His heartbeat began to increase and beads of cold sweat ran down his forehead. He became extremely nervous and suddenly felt his legs weaken at the knees. In the reflection of the dimly lit street he could see that the bundle of clothing contained the body of a dead woman. At the same time Cross heard other footsteps approaching, and more from fear than for any other reason, stepped back to hide in the shadows of a nearby doorway. As the footsteps came nearer he recognized their owner, a fellow market worker, John Paul.

Both men stood motionless in the darkness, staring at the body that lay on the pavement before them. Paul believed that the woman was still alive but very drunk. Cross thought otherwise and gathered up the strength to place his hand on the woman's cheek; it was still warm, but the body felt limp.

Fear started to overcome any thoughts of bravery, and Cross suggested they informed the police immediately. They hurriedly made their way towards the nearest police station and quickly reached Baker's Row a short distance away. There they met Police Constable Misen, who was patrolling his beat. The two men excitedly told him of what they had found, and at first Misen looked at them somewhat sceptically, wondering whether they had been drinking.

Meanwhile, following the departure of Cross and Paul from where the body lay, Police Constable John Neil walked along Bucks Row, which was for that particular night part of his beat patrol. The street lighting was poor, with just a single gas lamp partially illuminating a warehouse standing on one side of the street. There was a row of terraced houses opposite on the other side. In a gap between the houses was a gateway which led to some stables. The gates were closed, but lying next to them on the pavement, he found the murdered woman. He could see from the light of his 'Bullseye' lamp that the body lay with one arm close to the stable gate and the other stretching outward across the pavement. Her throat had been cut from ear to ear. PC Neil had walked that part of his beat some 30 minutes earlier and knew that the body had not been there at that time. He was very shortly joined by PC Misen, in company with Cross and Paul.

Doctor Rees Ralph Llewellyn was a divisional police surgeon who lived at his surgery at 152 Whitechapel Road, which was close to Bucks Row. He was aroused from his sleep by heavy banging on the door and knew instantly that it would be a man in uniform.

'There's been a murder in Bucks Row, doctor, they need you there quick.'

Llewellyn nodded and the officer stormed off.

It had been a misty, damp night, and as the doctor walked, bag in hand, towards the scene, he could feel a cold breeze that normally indicated daylight wasn't too far away. He made his way along Bucks Row and saw flashing lights coming from a small group of people now gathered around where the body lay. Llewellyn wondered for how long he would be needed and yearned for the bed he had just prematurely left.

The street lighting was poor and almost made it impossible for the police surgeon to carry out a full examination of the body. He asked PCs Misen and Neil to do the best they could with their lamps, before confirming that the woman was dead. He could see from his initial examination that the victim had an incision about 4 inches in length running from below the left side of the jaw, and another deeper cut just below this one. The second cut had in fact sliced through the throat back to the vertebrae, finishing about 3 inches below the right jaw. Llewellyn also found a wineglass near to where the body lay and handed it to one of the police officers. Although he observed that only half of the blood he would normally expect to find was present in the gutter, he was convinced that the victim had been murdered where she had been found. Nothing more could be revealed in the poor light available, and the doctor instructed the body to be removed to the Whitechapel Mortuary, where a more thorough examination could be made. Two police officers who had been sent to Bucks Row to assist Misen and Neil lifted the body from the pavement and saw that the clothing of the dead woman was saturated with blood. The small amount left in the gutter was later washed away by a local resident with a bucket of water.

The mortuary was situated next door to the local workhouse, and the body was accompanied by two police inspectors from Bethnal Green Police Station. Amazingly, there was some delay before the dead woman could be further examined for evidence, because of the stubborn demands of two workhouse inmates who wanted to finish their breakfasts before starting the day's routine chores. When the officers eventually began to remove the victim's clothing, they were the first to see loops of bowel penetrating from the abdomen, a sight which quite horrified them.

Dr Llewellyn carried out a full post-mortem examination and reported the following:

> *Several jagged incisions had ripped the abdomen open down its full length and there were two stab wounds in the genitals. In addition to the cut throat, there were bruises on the right side of the jaw, possibly due to pressure exerted by gripping fingers.*

The doctor believed that the mutilations might have been caused by a left-handed person, using a long-bladed knife. From the temperature taken between her legs Llewellyn was able to say that the victim had been dead for approximately half an hour. *There was no motive to the murder*.

Initial enquiries made to trace the identity of the dead woman met with some difficulties. A number of women who thought they could identify the body failed to do so after attending the mortuary during the day. The name of a workhouse in Lambeth was found stamped on one of the victim's petticoats. From that, Police Inspector Helson learned that the dead woman was known to residents in Thrawl Street, Spitalfields. Initially the officer could only find out that she was known to most people as 'Polly'. However, he persisted with his enquiries, and the victim was eventually named as Mary Ann Nichols, a 42-year-old prostitute. Her husband, William Nichols, later formally identified the body as being his wife, after the coroner's inquest had been opened.

Police officers quickly traced a friend of the dead woman, another prostitute, Emily 'Nelly' Holland. She had previously shared a room with Nichols and four other women at 18 Thrawl Street. Holland told them that she had spoken to Mary Nichols at about 2.30 a.m., one hour before the murder had been committed, on the corner of Osborn Street and Brick Lane. When first interviewed, she became very distressed and found it difficult to accept the nature of the atrocities Mary had been subjected to. Nichols had told Holland that she had earned her rent money 'twice over' that day and spent it in drink in the Frying Pan public house. In between her tears Emily told officers, *'When I saw her, she was wearing a black straw bonnet. She told me what a jolly bonnet she had and that she would soon get her doss money for the night.'* She had tried to persuade her friend to go with her, but Nichols had told her, *'I can't, I'm expected in a doss-house in Flower Dean Street where they sleeps men as well as women.'* Holland also explained that poor wretched Mary was extremely drunk, although *'Polly appeared confident she could raise the extra money for her bed.'* That was the last time Mary Ann Nichols was seen alive and the site where Emily Holland had spoken to her was less than half a mile away from where her body was later found.

Detective Inspector Frederick Abberline from Scotland Yard was appointed as the Senior Investigating Officer to lead a team of CID officers to investigate the murder. He soon discovered that the initial impact on the local community was one of shock, and not much information was forthcoming. People discussed the murder in whispers on street corners and in public houses. At first, stories were told of local protection gangs, 'Victorian-type pimps', who were 'looking after prostitutes for money'. But when prostitutes failed to pay their protection money they were beaten up. People spread gossip about earlier East End killings and tried to link the murder of Mary Nichols to those. None of this information made Abberline's task an easy one.

At the inquest that followed, Inspector Joseph Henry Helson, who was stationed at Bethnal Green Police Station at the time of the murder, told the coroner and the packed courtroom audience,

> '*I first got the news of the murder at 6.45 and went to the mortuary after 8. The woman's stays had prevented further wounds being caused above the level of the diaphragm and the abdominal wounds had been caused while the body was still dressed. None of the petticoats or skirts were torn.*'

The inquest into the death was adjourned on several occasions awaiting further developments, but the outcome was soon to be overtaken by other events.

Nichols – An Hypothesis, One Hundred Years On

If the murder of Mary Nichols happened today the Senior Investigating Officer, referred to as the SIO, would be a detective superintendent who was either responsible for the management of crime in the Whitechapel area or one posted to a central location in the force area, specializing in murder and other serious crime investigations. The Senior Investigating Officer in this case is to be Detective Superintendent Frederick Abberline.

The news of this particular murder would have been relayed to Abberline without delay. His first priority should then have been to immediately order preservation of the scene, leaving the body intact and where it was found. He would also have requested for a rendezvous point to be identified near the scene for other officers and experts to meet – this avoids unnecessary disturbance of the area around the body by people attending to complete specific functions.

The Senior Investigating Officer would then look towards the individual skill areas of those people he required to assist during the initial stages of the investigation. Scenes of crime officers are a mixture of police and civilian employees, highly trained in crime scene examination. Their responsibilities include searching for, recovering and preserving evidence. They are supported by facilities such as Forensic Science laboratories and Fingerprint Identification services.

In the majority of cases a coroner's officer is a civilian, usually employed by a police authority to assist local coroners in matters such as post-mortem arrangements, inquests and liaison between police and other agencies, including victims or families of victims. For a senior investigating officer dealing with a crime of murder, the coroner's officer can be of valuable assistance in making necessary arrangements for Home Office pathologists to conduct post mortems, and for reporting details of murders and suspicious deaths to the coroner responsible for the area in which the death has occurred.

In recent years a number of police forces have developed 'Intelligence Cells' to support major criminal investigations. Police officers and civilian support staff, specially trained in areas of intelligence, work together to evaluate and analyse information connected with the investigation. Intelligence analysts are civilian operatives, highly trained in Crime Pattern Analysis, a method of identifying patterns of crime committed across a particular geographical area. They can also be professional profilers responsible for compiling antecedent facts relative to a victim of crime and on occasions, suspected offenders. A suspect's identity does not necessarily need to be known to complete a profile. One piece of information that comes to the knowledge of the police may indicate the kind of person the offender is, and when added to other intelligence, a picture of the character of the person responsible for the crime can emerge. A few intelligence analysts are also qualified in the development of Psychological Profiles, which are primarily aimed towards identifying the mental condition of an offender.

Having identified those specialist skills required, Abberline could then have asked for the following individuals to attend at the designated rendezvous point as soon as possible:

1. The first police officer who arrived at the scene and saw the body, so that the Senior Investigating Officer could obtain first-hand information as to what had been observed initially.

2. A deputy senior investigating officer, usually of the rank of detective chief inspector, to assist and support Abberline.

3. A coroner's officer to inform the local coroner of the circumstances and to arrange for a post mortem to take place when required.

4. A police surgeon to formally certify death.

5. A police photographer, who would have the responsibility of photographing the scene.

6. Scenes of crime officers to arrange a detailed examination of the scene and to ensure that a video recording was made for future reference.

7. A small number of uniformed police officers to assist with scene preservation. One officer would be nominated to maintain a log or record of people attending the scene together with their times of arrival and departure.

8. An intelligence officer to obtain first-hand knowledge and liaise with the Senior Investigating Officer for the purposes of setting up an Intelligence Cell if required.

At the commencement of the investigation, the following areas would be considered.

The Scene

One of the first requirements for a senior investigating officer is to select an area for detailed examination which surrounds the location where the body was found. This would then be formally known as the 'murder scene' and is usually identified by the SIO after consultation with other experts. The murder scene would then be cordoned off at its extremities with tape, usually marked with the words 'Police Line – Do Not Cross'. In this case either the whole of Bucks Row would be treated as the scene, or 100 yards either side of where the body was found, whichever was the shortest distance. Although the stable gates near to where the victim lay were closed, the entrance which led to the inside of the stables would be included as part of the scene.

In the majority of cases it is preferable to make early decisions as to which direction the investigation should be steered. Before doing so, Abberline would need to establish two major factors. Firstly, the cause of death and how the victim died, and secondly, any apparent reason for the murder to have been committed. There are a number of possible motives to be considered according to circumstances. However, before a decision is made, consideration should be given to any evidence supporting a motive of theft, robbery, sexual intentions or an incident of a domestic nature, such as revenge or pure hatred against the victim.

In cases where a motive or reason for a murder cannot be identified, the subsequent investigation has to be focused on a much wider plain than in circumstances where they are known. The Lines of Enquiry that drive an investigation forward need only concentrate on those investigative areas that are fundamental to the motive. Where there has been a failure to identify a reason behind a crime, then some difficulties could arise for a senior investigating officer. The wider the areas to be investigated, the greater the risk of unimportant issues clouding the fundamental factors that do exist.

It is essential that items of evidential value found at the scene be identified and recovered as quickly as possible. The first problem to be overcome by the Senior Investigating Officer is the fact that within a short period of time, people would be leaving their terraced houses in Bucks Row to go to work, or stopping inquisitively to look at what was happening. Police officers would need to be deployed to ensure free passage for residents, with minimal disturbance being caused to the scene.

Having consulted with the police surgeon, Doctor Llewellyn, and having confirmed that a weapon was used, Abberline would obtain an initial description of the knife used by the killer, no matter how vague that description would be. Directions would then be given for police officers to commence a fingertip search of the street area within the scene parameters, followed by a detailed search of alleyways and backs of premises. If daylight was not imminent, then floodlighting would be introduced to assist the search teams.

After arranging for the body and surrounding area to be photographed and video recorded, scenes of crime officers would be instructed to thoroughly examine the scene and take samples of any blood or other human traces found. In addition, any fibres or other articles discovered that could have belonged to the victim or killer, would be later handed to a police officer who is specially trained and known as the 'Exhibits Officer', who would then be responsible for recording and monitoring any such items recovered.

At this stage Abberline would have to decide whether or not a Forensic Team would be required to attend. His decision would depend upon whether he thought that scientists should recover the samples personally and before laboratory analysis. The alternative and most common practice is for a scenes of crime officer to recover and arrange the transfer of any samples to the laboratory for later examination. There are occasions when it is preferable for a scientist to participate in scene examination. For example, should a fingerprint impression in blood have been left by an offender, there are two options for the Senior Investigating Officer to consider. The blood in which the impression has been made could be recovered and taken back to the laboratory for analysis. If that were to be the case, then the fingerprint impression would probably be destroyed during the recovery process and lose its evidential value. If the impression was transferred away from the scene for searching and identification purposes, then the blood would be corrupted and valueless. In those circumstances a senior investigating officer would normally consult with a scientist as to which course of action would be of more evidential value, and request that the forensic expert assists with the recovery of the sample.

Where circumstances dictate that the introduction of a forensic examination would not be more beneficial than a thorough examination by scenes of crime officers, then the exercise would be pointless. If, however, the scene could provide evidence that could only be obtained forensically, then the attendance at the scene of a team of scientists would become the favoured option. Scenes that are contained inside premises usually require forensic examination because the recovery of evidence sometimes requires walls and floors to be forensically treated. If the decision made by the Senior Investigating Officer is not to prefer a scientific examination, then any article or item recovered could still be submitted for forensic examination at a later date. An officer, preferably with experience in scene examination, would also be nominated as the 'Scene Manager', whose primary responsibility would be to ensure that the Senior Investigating Officer's wishes were carried out efficiently.

The coroner's officer would be asked to arrange a post mortem of the body as soon as possible by a Home Office pathologist. A request could also be made for the pathologist to attend and view the body in the position it was found. Only when this stage had been reached would the body of the victim be removed to the mortuary for further examination.

Detective officers would be directed to make initial enquiries and obtain names and addresses of potential witnesses who would be interviewed in depth at a later time. The two witnesses, Cross and Paul, would be transferred to the nearest police station for full written statements to be obtained from them as soon as possible. Arrangements would also be made for PCs Misen and Neil to be interviewed by detective officers and make formal statements. Until a motive was established, all witnesses' evidence would be carefully scrutinized and corroboration would be sought to verify their stories.

The Post Mortem

When satisfied that the scene had been secured and arrangements made for the necessary examinations to take place, Abberline would then attend a post mortem on the victim. The need for such an examination might appear obvious to the observer, but there are a number of fundamental issues that would need to be addressed.

The pathologist would attempt to identify the cause of death, which in Mary Nichols' case was heart failure due to a loss of blood caused by the cutting of the windpipe. Further examination could also reveal whether or not the victim

13

suffered from any other illness that could have eventually caused death or, more importantly, could have contributed towards it. In this case there were none.

The presence of bruises on the right side of the jaw would indicate that the killer needed to grab and restrict his victim prior to cutting her throat. That could help to confirm that the neck wound was the first and fatal wound inflicted. It could also indicate to Abberline that Nichols was already dead when she was subjected to further violence. Each individual injury found to have been sustained during the examination would be carefully photographed, for further viewing later.

From the nature of the injuries on the body, it is possible for a pathologist to create an accurate description of the weapon used, or to identify a number of features, such as, the weapon was a knife which had a long, narrow blade. The angle of entry and the features surrounding the cuts made to the victim indicated that the killer was left-handed. Those were the important facts established in the Nichols case.

The nature of the injuries could also provide Abberline with important information. For example, where the murderer's knife had entered the body, there could be one site of entry through the broken outer skin. However, beneath the outer flesh there could be several wounds, each representing a different direction in which the murder weapon had travelled. This could confirm that once the killer had stabbed his victim, he then made a 'sawing' action before fully removing the knife from the body. Those facts would assist the Senior Investigating Officer in determining the state of the killer's mind when committing the crime and in establishing whether or not it was a frenzied attack. When considering the mental attitude of the killer, Abberline would observe the cutting open of the abdomen and could draw inferences which might lead him to believe that the attack upon Nichols was a frenzied one, rather than a controlled deliberate mutilation.

14

The nature of a killer's mind often falls into two categories. Firstly, the frenzied attack, which results from fear or hatred and which if spontaneous, is usually quite different from the second category, in which a controlled approach stems from a desire by the attacker to be in complete control and have power over the victim. These factors would be important to Abberline when trying to establish a motive. In the case of Mary Nichols, the clues obtained from the post mortem would support a belief that the attack was of a frenzied nature. The problem facing both Abberline and Llewellyn would be establishing the reasons for the two stab wounds to the victim's genitals. These injuries could have been part of the frenzied and excited attack, or could justifiably be recognized as a positive sign of a sexual deviance being present in the attacker's character.

At this stage of the investigation there appear to be more factors supporting the theory that the killer, at the time, was in a frenzied state of mind, rather than embellishing the theory that the motive had sexual connotations. However, the presence of human semen might not necessarily have been sought because, as in the case of blood, semen was not considered important in assisting with the identification of an offender in 1888.

There are occasions at post mortems when the Senior Investigating Officer and pathologist confidentially share information resulting from the examination of the body, which may not be disclosed to any other person, including members of the Investigation Team. Such restricted information, if withheld, could later be used to assist the SIO in positively identifying the murderer and perhaps be of some evidential value once the killer has been identified. Such action could also help in the elimination of suspects or individuals who confess to murders for their own reasons. For example, disclosure of information known only to the Senior Investigating Officer, pathologist and the killer, by a person interviewed as a suspect, could be vital in later securing a conviction.

In the case of Mary Nichols, details of the kind of murder weapon used would be widely publicized because of the need for assistance in its recovery. The way in which she died might also be openly disclosed, because of the necessity to warn the public to be wary of the type of person the police were seeking to trace. This action would not necessarily be for their own protection, but to hopefully gain public support to supply information.

The belief that the murderer was left-handed could be chosen as information not to be divulged to any other person other than the Senior Investigating Officer and pathologist.

The Investigation Set-up

Major Incident Rooms are primarily set up for the purposes of recording, evaluating and analysing information. There are two kinds, one which is supported by a computerized database, and the other a manual card-index system, which serves the same purpose, but for obvious reasons is not so effective as that supported by a computerized system. There is little doubt that the murder of Mary Nichols would justify the opening of a Major Incident Room supported by information technology, which would be sited at a predetermined location, preferably within easy reach of the scene and witnesses.

Following the post mortem, Detective Superintendent Abberline would visit the Major Incident Room, usually referred to as the MIR, to review the situation and further structure his investigation. Staff would already have been chosen and given the responsibility of setting up the MIR under the management of a senior police officer, usually of detective inspector rank, referred to as the 'Office Manager', whose role entails being responsible for dealing with all issues, both administratively and operationally, that are relevant to the running of the Major Incident Room. The Office Manager would be accountable

16

directly to Abberline. The selected personnel to work in the Major Incident Room would comprise indexers and inputters, usually a mix of civilians and police officers who possess detailed knowledge of the management of the database. Statement readers, usually detective sergeants, would also be nominated for the task of scrutinizing every witness statement, obtaining and highlighting important pieces of information that require further investigation.

It would then be the responsibility of the Senior Investigating Officer and his or her deputy to take stock and analyse the information already in their possession. In the case of Mary Nichols, the following facts would be accepted:

1. The intention of the suspect was to kill his victim, due to the ferocity of the attack.

2. The victim was a known female prostitute.

3. The offence took place during the hours of darkness and the scene was extremely obscure, offering a cloak beneath which the killer could commit the crime without being seen.

4. A knife with a long, narrow blade had been used to commit the offence.

5. The body had received stab wounds in addition to lacerations.

6. There was no apparent motive, although sexual connotations did exist because of the victim being stabbed in the genitals.

7. The victim had been manhandled around the throat prior to death, evidenced by the fingermark bruises.

8.   The degree of violence used against the victim was extreme, far more than was needed to cause death, the result being a frenzied attack probably occurring after death.

Following a detailed examination of the facts relevant to the murder and circumstances in which Nichols met her death, Abberline would then have to decide upon the Lines of Enquiry he required to direct the investigation during the initial stages. It is suggested that the following areas would be chosen for investigative work to be completed:

1. *The Scene*
A thorough and professional search by trained scenes of crime officers or forensic scientists is essential during the initial stages of a murder investigation. The details of any items recovered would be given to the Major Incident Room Exhibits Officer for recording purposes, and the results of forensic examinations and enquiries made known to the Senior Investigating Officer. The scene would not be disturbed or returned to normality until the experts had concluded their examination and were fully satisfied nothing remained that could be important to the investigation. During all this time, the scene would remain secure with the physical presence of a police officer.

The wineglass recovered at the scene by Dr Llewellyn would be handed to the Exhibits Officer who, after making an appropriate record, would then submit the item for fingerprint examination through the Scenes of Crime Department.

2. *House to House Enquiries*
A residential area surrounding the murder scene in Bucks Row would be identified as possibly housing witnesses who could assist the enquiry. Police officers under the supervision of a specially trained sergeant would be given the task of calling at

houses and places of employment. The officers would be briefed as to what questions would be asked of householders and other occupiers, to elicit appropriate responses for evidence and information-gathering. Individuals could be asked about their whereabouts between 10.00 p.m. and 6.00 a.m. during the night of the murder and whether or not they heard or saw anything or any person acting suspiciously. Each officer would be given a questionnaire to complete, and details of any person in possession of information thought to be important to the investigation would be passed on for a detective officer to revisit at a later time and obtain a full statement.

3. The Victim

A full antecedent history of the victim would be compiled and would include information of any known relatives and associates. Details of the last time Nichols was seen alive, by whom and where, would also be contained within the Victim's Profile, including any financial or other domestic problems she may have had. The objective of this exercise is twofold. Firstly, the obtaining of historical and detailed information of the victim could lead to the early recognition of a suspect or suspects, together with a possible motive for the murder. Secondly, such a profile could assist in briefing operational officers, who would need to be aware of the victim's background to assist them with their enquiries.

4. The Suspect or Offender

Suspect or Offender Profiles, which contain similar information to that contained in the Victim Profile, would include any person known to the victim who could have a reason for committing the murder. Details of individuals identified as potential suspects by members of the public or other sources of information would also be recorded. Searches of police records with a view to identifying individuals who had committed crimes of a similar *modus operandi* would be completed, although it would be doubtful that any such person would be at liberty. As much detail as possible would be collected together to give personal backgrounds to assist officers responsible for interviewing those thought to have been involved in the murder. One other advantage in completing an Offender Profile could be the assistance it would give to the Senior Investigating Officer in identifying individuals who could not be readily eliminated from the investigation, by comparing their backgrounds with that of the suspect.

5. Mental Hospitals
Because of the nature of the attack on Mary Nichols and the absence of any motive, local mental institutions would normally be visited, with a view to tracing and eliminating any patient who could have been absent at the time of the murder. Included in this category would also be general hospitals, where enquiries would be made to trace any person who may have sought treatment for injuries possibly received during the attack on the victim.

6. Crime Pattern Analysis
In addition to the Major Incident Room, an Intelligence Cell could be created, in which police and civilian personnel would be tasked with processing information thought to be relevant to the investigation. Included in the cell would be an intelligence analyst, who would be responsible for enquiring into and analysing similar attacks on women that might have occurred elsewhere and prior to the Mary Nichols murder. The analyst would also assist with creating the Victim and Suspect Profiles.

7. *Press and Media*

An essential facility for the Senior Investigating Officer, to make appeals for assistance from the public and circulate information aimed towards maintaining public interest in the case. A press officer would be appointed to deal with enquiries from the media and a press conference, usually chaired by the SIO, would be held within 12 hours of the murder being discovered. It is necessary for the senior officer to be left free from unnecessary interruptions and allowed to concentrate on the investigation, therefore, after the initial press conference has been held, the usual practice is for the nominated press officer to continue liaison with the media.

There would be three additional Lines of Enquiry, nominated by Abberline, which would be given top priority.

8. *Wineglass Recovered at Scene*

Because of the obvious importance attached to this particular item, it would be treated separately from the Line of Enquiry associated with the scene examination. The glass would be preserved for fingerprint and forensic examination, and Abberline would request that the results be made known to him as soon as possible.

9. *Frying Pan Public House*

The premises were situated in Thrawl Street at the corner with Brick Lane. Because of the information provided by the witness Holland, that the deceased woman appeared to have spent most of the previous day there, enquiries would be needed to ascertain a number of factors. These would include answers to the following questions:

a) How long did Nichols spend in the premises during the previous 24 hours?
b) Who was she seen to be associating with?

c) Were there any strangers in the premises at the same time Nichols was there?

d) How many witnesses can verify seeing Nichols there?

e) What was her association with the public house? Was she a regular customer or did she just pay occasional visits there?

f) Had she had any disagreements with any other person recently?

10. The Black Straw Bonnet Belonging to the Victim
It is apparent from what the witness Holland told the police, that Nichols had only recently come into possession of the item. Enquiries would be needed to ascertain where she obtained the bonnet from. There could be a possibility that the killer gave it to her. For that reason, it would be submitted for forensic examination together with the remainder of the victim's clothing.

Having identified the Lines of Enquiry, Abberline would then choose his Management Team. This would consist of police officers and civilians who would have responsibility for the management of those individual Lines of Enquiry already identified. An administration and finance officer would also be included on the team, to assist the Senior Investigating Officer in welfare, resource and budgetary matters.

The SIO also makes decisions on hours of working for those persons seconded to the investigation and upon the regularity of daily briefings and debriefings. It is common practice for the senior officer to meet the Management Team at least once a day, and that meeting should be followed by a full briefing of all personnel to update everyone on how the investigation is progressing.

Mary Ann Nichols – Areas to be examined

At the first meeting of his Management Team, Detective Superintendent Abberline would identify the Lines of Enquiry for which each member would be responsible. Other issues to be discussed would include the numbers of police officers and civilian or support staff that would be required for investigation and administration purposes. Every decision made would be recorded in a Policy File, copies of which would be inputted onto the computer system and maintained for future reference.

When satisfied that the Management Team was fully aware of individual responsibilities and how the investigation was to be directed, the meeting would then possibly discuss a number of fundamental issues that existed. The following questions could be asked by those present:

1. Had the victim been killed at the scene where she had been found?

2. What was the precise time of death?

3. Were there any witnesses to the murder?

4. Were there any other crimes committed in the immediate area of the crime?

5. Were there any known associates of the victim?

6. Was there any knowledge of mentally disturbed persons frequenting the area having absconded or being absent from a hospital or institution?

7. Were there any other similar murders committed elsewhere in the country?

1. Had the victim been killed at the scene where she had been found?

A number of issues would have to be addressed to confirm whether or not the scene of the crime was actually where the body was found. For instance, where there is an absence of blood either at the scene or remaining inside the body, then the victim could have been murdered elsewhere and carried to the location where she lay. Therefore the volume of blood found on the floor directly beneath, or in the immediate vicinity of where the body was, should have been compared with the amount left inside her body. The amounts of blood remaining in the body would be determined at the subsequent post mortem. A good yardstick for such comparison is that an average person has approximately one pint of blood for every stone in weight.

Information from witnesses could assist in confirming where the victim had been attacked and murdered. Suspicious sounds and noises overheard at the time Nichols was believed to have died would be important. Although there is little doubt that she was attacked and killed at the place where her body was found, signs of violence in that immediate vicinity would support that belief.

2. What was the precise time of death?

The temperature of a body following death gives some indication as to when the victim died. The colder the temperature of the victim, then the more time had elapsed between death and the initial examination. At 4.00 a.m. Dr Llewellyn was of the opinion that the woman had been dead for approximately 30 minutes which would have put her death at 3.30 a.m.

The last sighting of the victim alive would assist Abberline to identify a period of time during which the murder had taken place. Witnesses hearing or seeing the attack could also assist from their evidence in determining the time of death.

3. Were there any witnesses to the murder?

Numerous people living in the neighbourhood of Bucks Row were interviewed by police officers, but the majority stated that they hadn't heard or seen anything that would be useful to the investigation. Those that did gave evidence that was slightly conflicting. Harriet Lilley, who lived just two doors away from where Nichols' body was found, told police officers that she and her husband had been awakened at 3.30 a.m. on the morning of the murder and heard whispering in the street outside. The whispering was then followed by the sounds of gasps and moans, but both Lilley and her husband returned to sleep. However, Patrick Mulshaw informed the inquest that he had been standing near to the murder scene, smoking. He was employed as a nightwatchman at premises in the same vicinity, and hadn't seen or heard anything between 2.30 a.m. and 3.30 a.m.

Emily Holland, who knew the victim, stated that she had seen Nichols at about 2.30 a.m. in Osborn Street in a very drunken state. Nichols stopped to tell her that she still had to earn enough money to pay for her night's bed, before staggering away. Osborn Street was approximately half a mile away from where the victim's body was later found. There is no doubt that Holland was the last person to see Nichols alive, apart from the killer.

4. Were any other crimes committed in the immediate area of the crime?

There have been many instances when criminals have committed serious acts of violence whilst leaving the scene of another less serious crime such as burglary, robbery or theft. In most cases the violence has been used to effect an escape.

Enquiries into other possible offences being committed prior to or after the commission of the murder were not made. However, in circumstances where the murder weapon has not been recovered, the possibility of the item having come into the killer's possession during the course of another crime is a real one, although unlikely in the Nichols case. The type of weapon used in this murder and the likelihood of it being used again in other murders that followed, made such a possibility unlikely. If a screwdriver had been used or another heavy instrument had delivered fatal blows to the victim's head, then perhaps stronger consideration could have been given to the possibility that the weapon might have been used in other, less serious crimes.

5. *Were there any known associates of the victim?*

Following the breakdown of her marriage, Mary Ann Nichols spent most of her time during the last eight years of her life in workhouses, the last one being the Mitcham Workhouse in Holborn, before she was employed by the Cowdry family in April 1888. She was known to many people throughout the East End of London because of the nature of her employment. Police officers compiling the Victim's Profile should have been searching for an associate with a motive for killing the victim. No such person was traced in this case.

6. *Was there any knowledge of mentally disturbed persons frequenting the area and/or having absconded from a hospital or institution?*

Enquiries made were met with a negative result.

7. *Were there any other similar murders committed else-where in the country?*

In Victorian England news travelled slowly across the country. Details of similar atrocities committed outside the London area may not have been available to Scotland Yard. As a result of the introduction of information technology to support Police Intelligence, that problem would not exist today. However, there is little doubt that details of similar murders to that of the Ripper would have eventually come to the notice of the murder investigation team.

In addition to the police networked databases, the capability of the current press and media to circulate news nationally and internationally is far greater and more effective than it was in 1888. The police service of today has an extremely efficient internal communications system, which did not exist a hundred years ago.

Two

Annie May Chapman

*'There lying at the foot of the steps which led into the backyard
was the body of a woman with her throat cut'*

Annie May Chapman was an attractive, well-proportioned
woman in her mid-forties. She had two children from a
previous marriage to Fred Chapman, who was a soldier living
in barracks near Windsor Castle before leaving the Army and
taking up employment as a coachman. One of the children, a
son, was severely deformed at birth and lived his life in a home
for cripples, which caused Annie great distress. All that is
known about the other child is that she was a girl and, it is said,
resided in an institution somewhere in France.

Annie and Fred Chapman parted company some years prior
to her death. A number of stories were told at the time, some
concerning other soldiers going with Annie, but it would appear
that both husband and wife fell upon hard times and a number
of family pressures resulted in the separation. After leaving
Fred Chapman, she lived with a man who made wire sieves for
a short while, before maintainance payments made by her
husband ceased and life became intolerable. Her last place of
lodgings was at 35 Dorset Street in Whitechapel, apparently an
habitual abode for thieves, rogues, vagabonds and prostitutes. It
was known locally as Crossingham's Common Lodging-House.

The deputy manager was Timothy Donovan, who used to charge fourpence for a bed for the night. Annie Chapman frequently paid eightpence for the luxury of having a double bed for herself. Whether that was to accommodate clients is not known.

At 1.45 a.m. on Saturday, 8 September 1888, Donovan found Annie Chapman sitting in the kitchen of his lodging-house. She was eating a baked potato and appeared to be very dejected and exhausted. When asked if she was going to bed, Annie replied that she had no money and despite her previous custom, the deputy manager reminded her of the rules of the house, 'No money, no bed'. A disillusioned Annie Chapman was forced to leave 35 Dorset Street to search for money to pay for a bed for that night.

Hanbury Street was less than half a mile from Bucks Row, the scene of the first murder. There were a large number of three-storey houses which had originally been built for the purposes of accommodating local workers. As time went by, the majority of dwellings became common lodging-houses. In September 1888 there were 17 people lodging at number 29. The house was entered by a front door which led to a passageway allowing access to either the stairs or a yard at the rear. It was common practice to leave both the front and rear doors unlocked, providing opportunities for local prostitutes to take their clients into the backyard to conduct their business.

At 6.00 a.m. each morning it was customary for John Davis, who occupied the third floor front room at 29 Hanbury Street with his wife and three sons, to get up and make his way to work. He was employed as a carman in Leadenhall Market and had been lodging at the Hanbury Street address for approximately two weeks. Saturday, 8 September 1888, was no exception, and with tiredness still in his eyes Davis made his way downstairs, where he noticed that the back door was closed. He stood at the bottom of the stairs for a while, stretching himself and trying to come to terms with the day's work that lay in front of him. He was an orderly type of person and, to him, seeing the back door closed was unusual. He yawned as he walked down the hallway to open the door, not really thinking why it was closed in the first place. As he pushed it open he witnessed a scene that was to remain in his memory for the rest of his life. He started to weaken and gasped for air as he looked down upon a woman with her throat cut, lying at the foot of the steps leading into the backyard. The awesome sight brought Davis to his full senses, and panic then followed the initial shock. He fled from the house to seek help.

On the opposite side of the street to number 29 was a packing-case manufacturers by the name of Bayley's, and it was there that Davis sought refuge. Two night workers, James Kent and James Green, were looking forward to the end of their shift and saw the horror on Davis' pale face as he ran inside the building. In between gasps and stutters he told them what he had seen. At first both men found it difficult to accept what they had been told and stood looking expressionless at each other. Davis collapsed into a sitting position on top of a number of cardboard boxes. For a short time Green and Kent discussed what they should do. There was no one else in the building at Bayley's, so the two men decided to go with Davis to where he had seen the body. At first the frightened man was reluctant and petrified, but finally agreed. All three walked slowly and anxiously across the street to the backyard of the lodging-house.

It was still dark, but the men could see enough detail of the disturbing picture for them to appreciate what had happened. There was little doubt that the woman was dead and had been brutally murdered. Fear began to grip them, and they agreed that the police should be told immediately. They left to run to the local police station in Commercial Street. Police Inspector

Joseph Chandler was walking into Hanbury Street when he was almost knocked to the ground by Davis, Green and Kent. They spurted out what they had seen and took the Inspector to number 29, where he found the front door still open. Chandler smartly made his way along the passageway to the backyard and soon confirmed everything the three men had told him.

The dead woman was lying on her back, with her legs drawn up and her knees wide apart. The face was turned to one side, bruised and swollen, and the tongue was protruding through the teeth. There was a silk scarf wrapped around the neck. The hands and legs were smeared with blood, and the head had almost been completely severed from the body. As seasoned and experienced as the Inspector believed he was, the sight distressed him, but he managed to steel himself and remain composed.

Medical evidence at the inquest revealed that the throat had not been cut but viciously slashed from ear to ear. Incisions from left to right had been made in the throat and back. There were also two clean cuts made on the left side of the spine, parallel with each other and separated by only half an inch. Those incisions had facilitated the removal of a kidney. Doctor George Bagster Phillips told the inquest that the cuts to Annie May Chapman, another known prostitute, had been made by *'a very sharp knife with a thin, narrow blade…such as a doctor would use for surgery'*. The same knife had been used to cut the throat as well as the abdomen, and the length of the blade would have been between 6 and 8 inches in length. It was also suggested that the wounds *'showed indications of anatomical knowledge'*. The body had been virtually disembowelled, with the uterus and its appendages removed, but surprisingly there was relatively little blood in the yard where it had been found. Part of the small intestine had been pulled over the left shoulder.

32

The Divisional Police Surgeon, Dr Phillips, was summoned, as were senior police officers, including Detective Inspector Abberline of Scotland Yard. Dr Phillips formally pronounced death and made a cursory examination of the body before requesting it be removed to the mortuary. Two brass rings which had been removed from the victim's fingers, together with a few pennies and a couple of farthings, were all laid out neatly at the foot of the body. It was later confirmed that they were the contents of the dead woman's pockets, which had been torn open. There were also a piece of muslin, a comb and a paper case found nearby. Close to the head of the corpse was part of an envelope bearing the seal of the Sussex Regiment on the reverse. On the front of the envelope was the letter 'M' and a franking mark, 'London, 28 Aug., 1888'. There were no signs of any struggle having taken place, and Dr Phillips believed that the victim had been alive when she first entered the yard. He was also of the opinion that the silk scarf around the victim's neck was in place before the throat was cut.

The police surgeon also found a leather apron soaked with water and lying near an outside tap. When the finding of the leather apron became public knowledge, the majority of people believed it belonged to the killer. This resulted in a number of police enquiries being made to eliminate individuals whose employment required them to wear leather aprons. In fact the nickname 'Leather Apron' was initially given to the killer, which resulted in a number of persons being arrested and interviewed, but later released.

During the preliminary stages of the investigation, police officers spoke to a man by the name of Cadosh who lived next door to 29 Hanbury Street. At about 5.15 a.m. on the morning of the murder, Cadosh had been in his backyard when he heard a voice say 'No', followed by the sound of someone falling against the fence. He did nothing and later stated that such sounds were commonplace in that part of the neighbour-hood.

A local newspaper carried the report of the murder as follows:

Ghastly Murder in the East End
Dreadful Mutilation of a Woman

Another murder of a character even more diabolical than that perpetrated in Buck's Row on Friday week, was discovered in the same neighbourhood on Saturday morning. At about six o'clock a woman was found lying in a backyard at the foot of a passage leading to a lodging-house in Old Brown's Lane, Spitalfields. The house is occupied by a Mrs Richardson, who lets it out to lodgers, and the door which admits to this passage, at the foot of which lies the yard where the body was found, is always open for the convenience of lodgers. A lodger named Davis was going down to work at the time mentioned and found the woman lying on her back close to the flight of steps leading into the yard. Her throat was cut in a fearful manner. The woman's body had been completely ripped open, and the heart and other organs laying about the place, and portions of the entrails round the victim's neck. An excited crowd gathered in front of Mrs Richardson's house and also round the mortuary in old Montague Street, whither the body was quickly conveyed. As the body lies in the rough coffin in which it has been placed in the mortuary – the same coffin in which the unfortunate Mrs Nichols was first placed – it presents a fearful sight. The body is that of a woman about 45 years of age. The height is exactly five feet. The complexion is fair, with wavy dark brown hair; the eyes are blue, and two lower teeth have been knocked out. The nose is rather large and prominent.

When Dr Phillips attended the mortuary later that day, at approximately 2.00 p.m., he complained that the body had been

34

undressed and washed down. The only article that had been left in place was the neckscarf tied around the victim's neck. Such practices had deprived the doctor of the opportunity to examine the blood flows with the injuries.

The results of the post mortem were deemed to be so horrific that at first they were not made public, but later appeared in *The Lancet*.

The throat had been cut from the left side of the neck with two distinct paralled incisions about half an inch apart. The abdomen had been entirely laid open and a bundle of the intestines severed from their mesenteric attachments. These had been scooped out of the abdomen and placed on the left shoulder of the prostrate woman, while from the pelvic region of the body the uterus with its ovaries, part of the vagina and a portion of the bladder had been cut out and entirely removed. Cause of death was ascertained as syncope or failure of the heart due to massive loss of blood from the cut throat.

The murdered woman was soon identified as Annie Chapman, a 45-year-old prostitute whose address was 35 Dorset Street.

One major question that puzzled the investigation team at the time, and still remains a mystery today, was how the killer made good his escape from an area which, at that time in the morning, was busy with market traders travelling to work. The police accepted that the person responsible must have possessed detailed knowledge of the local area to facilitate his escape, possibly by using side alleyways, backyards or gardens. The possibility that the murderer could have been dressed in working-class clothes to avoid looking conspicuous in that area was also considered. If that had been the case then the majority of early morning workers would, having just left the warmth of their beds, have walked to their workplaces with heads down looking towards the pavement. Any person passed in the street would probably have been greeted with 'Good morning' without attracting further attention.

Within days of Annie Chapman's murder the Senior Investigating Officer, Fred Abberline, arrested a man named William Henry Piggott following information received that Piggott had been seen in a public house, the Pope's Head in Gravesend, with bloodstains on his clothing. The matter was investigated by local police, and Piggott was initially interviewed by a police sergeant who confirmed that the suspect had injuries to both hands and appeared to be in a dazed state. Piggott also admitted being in Whitechapel on the Sunday following the murder. He told officers that he had received his injuries whilst trying to assist a woman who had fallen over in the street. According to Piggott, the woman had bitten him on his hand after he tried to assist her. He had struck the woman hard across the face and run off when he saw two police officers walking towards him. The amount of blood on Piggott's clothing was far more than that which would have come from the bite on his hand. There was never any explanation given, and the circumstances remain a mystery today. Piggott was eventually committed to an asylum after being declared insane.

On 26 September 1888, the coroner, Mr Baxter, stated the following:

The deceased entered the house in full possession of her faculties although with a very different object to her companion's. From the evidence which the condition of the yard afforded and the medical examination disclosed, it appeared that after the two had passed through the passage and opened the swing door at the end, they descended the three steps into the yard. The wretch must have then seized the deceased, perhaps with Judas-like approaches. He seized her by the chin. He pressed her throat, and while thus preventing the slightest cry, he at the same time produced insensibility and suffocation. There was no evidence of any struggle. The clothes were not torn. Even in those preliminaries the wretch seems to have known how to carry out efficiently his nefarious work. The deceased was then lowered to the ground and laid on her back, and although in doing so she may have fallen slightly against the fence, the movement was probably effected with care. Her throat was then cut in two places with savage determination, and the injuries of the abdomen commenced... The body had not been dissected but the injuries had been made by someone who had considerable anatomical skill and knowledge. There were no meaningless cuts... The organ had been taken by one who knew where to find it, what difficulties he would have to contend against, and how he should use his knife so as to abstract the organ without injury to it. No unskilled person could have known where to find it or have recognized it when it was found. For instance, no mere slaughterer of animals could have carried out these operations. It must have been someone accustomed to the post-mortem room... The conclusion that the desire was to possess the missing abdominal organ seemed overwhelming ... The amount missing would go into a breakfast cup, and had not the medical examination been of a thorough and searching character it might easily have been left unnoticed that there was any portion of the body which had been taken... The difficulty in believing that the purport of the murderer was the possession of the missing abdominal organ was natural.

The second murder was the turning point which saw increased pressure come from members of the local Whitechapel community to find the person responsible. Public knowledge of the details of Annie Chapman's death, and the way in which her killer had performed without being seen, helped to create a phantom type of character, stories of whom quickly swept through the London streets. Vigilance committees were formed and made demands upon Sir Charles Warren, the commissioner of the Metropolitan Police, to increase the number of police officers working in the Whitechapel area. Local tradesmen gathered together and volunteered rewards for the capture of the killer. One of those committees wrote to the Home Office enquiring about rewards and received the following reply:

> *I am directed by the Secretary of State to acknowledge receipt of your letter of 16th, with reference to the question of the offer of a reward for the discovery of the perpetrators of the recent murders in Whitechapel, and I am to inform you that had the Secretary of State considered the case a proper one for the offer of a reward, he would at once have offered one on behalf of the government, but that the practice of offering rewards for the discovery of criminals was discontinued some years ago, because experience showed that such offers of reward tended to produce more harm than good. And the Secretary of State is satisfied that there is nothing in the circumstances of the present case to justify a departure from this rule.*
>
> > *I am, Sir,*
> >
> > > *Your obedient servant*
> > >
> > > > *G Leigh Pemberton*

Chapman – An Hypothesis, One Hundred Years On

During the eight-day period between the murders of Mary Ann Nichols and Annie May Chapman, the major investigation team should have developed a good working relationship. Members of the Management Team would understand what was expected of them, and their communication links with the Senior Investigating Officer would have strengthened as the enquiries progressed. The Major Incident Room staff would now be fully updated, with information being inputted into the computer system as it was received. The operational units, the house to house and outside enquiry crews would also be fully aware of each other's responsibilities.

The samples taken from the scene of the Nichols murder should have been given top priority for the attention of the Forensic Science Laboratory staff, and the following results may well have been returned to the Senior Investigating Officer, Detective Superintendent Abberline:

1. 'Foreign fibres', recovered from the victim's clothing, were made of wool, possibly having come from a cloak or other heavy garment. Each fibre contained a natural black dye.

2. The footprint impression found near to where the victim lay had been made by a size 8 boot. The print contained a number of ridges which had been cut by hand into the leather towards the front of the sole. Such a practice is common amongst seamen who require additional adhesion when aboard ship.

3. All of the blood samples taken from the scene have been identified as belonging to the victim.

Upon hearing the news of Annie Chapman's murder, Abberline could have considered the possibility that the killer might well have remained in the area near to the scene. If that was the case, he would have requested a number of police officers be directed immediately to search and detain any person for questioning about their whereabouts during the previous three hours. Those officers could be assisted by Air Support, and the helicopter crew would be briefed and instructed to report details of any person seen hanging around in the locality of the murder. People have committed serious crimes and remained in the area to watch the police activity that has subsequently taken place.

One of the first priorities for the Senior Investigating Officer would be to decide whether or not the Chapman murder should be linked to the Nichols investigation. Abberline would also have introduced the same structure used for the first murder and would have requested the following people meet at a pre-selected rendezvous point near to the scene:

1. The first police officer to have arrived at the scene.

2. The police surgeon, to confirm death.

3. A police photographer.

4. A scenes of crime team.

5. A coroner's officer.

6. A small team of police officers to assist with scene preservation.

7. One designated officer to record arrivals and departures of persons visiting the scene.

8. A designated senior CID officer who would be independent from the Nichols murder enquiry. If the two investigations were not linked, that senior officer would be given the responsibility for managing the Chapman investigation as a separate incident.

9. The member of the Nichols Management Team responsible for directing the Intelligence Cell, to obtain information for

the benefit of the Nichols Management Team, if the two murders were eventually linked together.

The Scene

Abberline would identify the scene as including the building known as 29 Hanbury Street. He would also include the pavement outside the front of the house up to the gutter or beginning of the highway. The rear of the premises would include the whole of the backyard in which the body was discovered.

The complete scene would then be photographed and video recorded, and Abberline would instruct the photographer to pay special attention to those items of property found within the immediate vicinity of where the body lay. They would be photographed separately for future viewing.

At this stage Abberline would also consider obtaining the services of a police plan drawer, who could provide a detailed sketch or plan of the area surrounding Hanbury Street. The plan would show the position of the scene compared with other residential and non-residential properties, streets, alleyways and gardens. This could later assist with identifying an escape route used by the killer.

The Intelligence Manager would be given the task of researching both murders and identifying any evidence that might support the theory that the same person was responsible for the murders of Nichols and Chapman. He would be assisted by the Intelligence Analyst already assigned to the first murder.

The coroner's officer would be told to arrange a visit to the scene by a Home Office pathologist, preferably the same one who had been involved in the Nichols murder. This would facilitate comparisons being made of the injuries inflicted upon both victims.

Arrangements could be made at this stage to open a Major Incident Room, either in the same building or certainly near to where the one responsible for the Nichols investigation was sited.

Abberline would consider the options of scene examination by his own scenes of crime officers or by a team of forensic scientists. This included the house and enclosed passageway that led from Hanbury Street to the backyard. Because of this, there would be a greater possibility of fibres, tissues and other items of evidential value being present, than if the scene was outside in the open air. The Senior Investigating Officer would favour the forensic option and the scenes of crime officers would maintain a liaison and provide support to the scientists.

Since Forensic Science Laboratories were first set up by the Home Office in the late 1930s, a great deal of progress has been made in this field, including the discovery of Genetic Finger-printing or, as it is more commonly known, DNA Profiling. Such a facility is frequently used today to assist in identifying persons responsible for murders, sexual offences or other crimes where human tissues and fluids are left on the victim or at the scene. In cases where the police are satisfied that a number of crimes have been committed by a serial killer, the involvement of scientists could be extensive, and it is normal practice to attach a forensic scientist to the Major Incident Room. Abberline could request that such a person become a member of his Management Team, with the responsibility of liaising with the laboratory when required. The scientist would also be able to offer valuable information in a consultative capacity on subjects arising from the forensic examinations.

During the detailed examination of the scene, bloodstains were found on the fence situated in the backyard and near to where Chapman's head lay. According to the local press, one of the bloodstains was quite large in size and resembled arterial bleeding. If that was the case, then there could have existed a possibility that the victim's throat had been cut whilst she was lying on her back on the ground.

The Post Mortem

As with Mary Nichols, the throat had been cut twice and the heart stopped because of loss of blood from those injuries. The 'double cut' could have resulted from resistance put up by the victim prior to her death, but there is little doubt that Chapman, like Nichols, had died before her body had been subjected to the mutilations that followed the initial cuts to her throat.

Having observed the way in which Annie Chapman's body had been violated, Abberline would probably reconsider the mental state of the killer. The opening of the abdomen and the removal of the internal organs, some of which were placed on the victim's left shoulder, could be regarded as showing a degree of planning by the murderer. The violent acts were also committed deliberately and with purpose, as was the removal of the internal organs. The factors supporting the belief that Nichols had been subjected to a frenzied attack were not present in the Chapman murder. The second murder had been committed in a more calculated and controlled manner. These facts would assist with the development of the Psychological Profile of the offender, and a picture would now emerge of an individual who sought total control of his victim by cutting her throat before continuing with the more serious acts of violence. Although such actions might well provide clues as to the mental state of the killer, a motive could not yet be identified from the information obtained in 1888.

Any suspicions that the killer possessed some anatomical knowledge that went beyond that of a normal 'animal slaughterer' would encourage Abberline to open up a new Line of Enquiry to seek further information from members of the medical profession. A certain amount of sensitivity and security would have to be attached to whatever knowledge came from those enquiries, particularly if prominent members of such an elite group of people became under suspicion.

Details of the missing organs would also be restricted to the Senior Investigating Officer and the pathologist, again to assist with the elimination of suspects and the identification of the real killer.

The Investigation Set-up

Following the post mortem of Annie Chapman, Abberline would visit the new Major Incident Room set up to investigate the second murder. He would probably have sensed an air of excitement which usually accompanies the initial structuring of an incident room, with people racing from one side of the room to the other, conversing with each other and answering telephone calls as they attempt to organize themselves. The busiest time for incident room staff is during the initial stages of an investigation, and individual responsibilities and workloads are usually immense.

Abberline could then arrange for a meeting to take place between himself, the Intelligence Manager, the senior CID officer who attended the second murder scene, and the scenes of crime officers from both murders. The circumstances of the Nichols and Chapman incidents would be discussed and consideration given to the linking of both investigations. From the information available the following points would be referred to:

1. Both scenes were very close to each other, within walking distance.

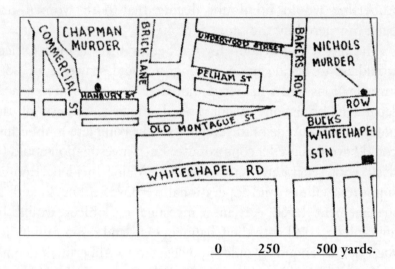

0   250   500 yards.

2. The murders occurred at similar times, both having been committed during the early hours of the morning.

3. Both crimes had been committed at locations which were extremely dark, reducing the possibility of the killer being seen.

4. Both victims were known common prostitutes and somewhat destitute.

5. A long, narrow-bladed knife had been used by the killer on both victims.

6. Both women had been subjected to severe violent acts, although the severity was greater in the Chapman case.

7. Both victims had their throats cut.

Charts outlining the sequence of events for both murders would be provided by the Intelligence Manager and Abberline would no doubt decide that both women had been murdered by the same person.

The next consideration for the Senior Investigating Officer would be to decide upon the logistics and structure of both investigations and whether or not they should be investigated separately or as one major linked enquiry. Because of the potential magnitude of the enquiries to be completed, Abberline could have favoured a compromise. Each investigation could be dealt with separately with individual Major Incident Rooms, support facilities and operational resources, but linked at management level. A senior investigating officer would be appointed to deal with the Chapman case, and responsibility for the Nichols enquiry would be delegated to Abberline's deputy. Abberline himself would overview both murders and provide the main link between the two newly appointed SIOs and their respective Management Teams.

The structure of the two investigations would contain a centralized Intelligence Cell, responsible for processing information relevant to both cases and under the management of a detective inspector. The Scenes of Crime support would be centralized, together with the press liaison officer. Such a structure would enable future murders committed by the same person to be investigated as satellites to the ongoing enquiries. Any requests for further support would be made directly to Abberline through the two newly appointed senior investigating officers. A contingency plan would be written by Abberline to deal with any future murder that was linked to the Nichols and Chapman cases.

Det. Supt. Abberline
(Overviewing Officer in Command)

Det. Chief Insp. (Nichols) **Det. Chief Insp.(Chapman)**
Sen. Investigating Officer **Sen. Investigating Officer**

Det. Inspector
(Liaison Officer)

Management Team **Management Team**

Intelligence Cell
(providing support to
each investigation)

Force Press Liaison Officer

Major Incident Room **Major Incident Room**

Scenes of Crime and
Forensic Scientists

Operational Crews **Operational Crews**

Having created the management structures for both murder investigations, Abberline would offer assistance to the Senior Investigating Officer now responsible for the Chapman murder. Certain facts obtained from initial observations would be as follows. Those factors present in both murders are marked with an asterisk.

1. The intention of the suspect was to kill his victim. *

2. The victim was a known female prostitute. *

3. The offence took place during the hours of darkness, limiting the possibility of detection by the murderer. *

4. A 'long, narrow-bladed knife' had been used to kill the victim. *

5. The scene was dark but overlooked by terraced houses.

6. The victim had probably walked voluntarily through a private passageway inside a house in Hanbury Street which led to a backyard.

7. The victim was found lying on her back with her knees bent upwards. *

8. The throat had been 'viciously slashed from ear to ear'. *

9. There was a possibility that the killer had some anatomical knowledge.

10. There was relatively little blood at the scene. The body could have been taken there after death, although unlikely.

11. The victim's clothing had been searched and the contents left at the scene in a neat pile.

12. There was no apparent motive. *

13. The degree of violence used was excessive. *

14. The killer managed to leave the scene without being seen. *

The next priority for Abberline would be to assist in deciding those Lines of Enquiry which would initially direct the Chapman investigation.

1. The Scene
Unlike the Nichols murder, Abberline requested a full forensic examination of the scene. This decision would have been made with the knowledge that 29 Hanbury Street could have offered clues as to the killer's identity, knowing that he had actually entered the premises to gain access to the backyard. Any part of the house known to have come into contact with the murderer or victim, including the passageway, would be subjected to forensic examination.

2. House to House Enquiries
A small residential area surrounding the murder scene and thought to contain possible witnesses would be identified and perhaps later extended if the initial enquiries were completed without success.

3. Area Search
Teams of police officers would be tasked with fingertip searches through an identified area surrounding the scene. The objective would be to recover the murder weapon or any other item dropped accidentally or discarded by the killer.

4. Cabs and Hansoms
Enquiries would be made to ascertain whether or not any person had been transported into the area surrounding Hanbury Street before or at the time of the murder. Details of any such person including a description would be obtained for elimination purposes.

49

5. Members of the Medical Profession

As a result of the allegations made that the killer could have possessed some anatomical knowledge, members of the medical profession would be interviewed. Initially, those enquiries would be restricted to private-practice doctors resident locally, and then extended to hospitals and institutions. The assistance and support of senior managers in the medical profession would be sought, and any information obtained would be treated in strictest confidence.

6. Hospital Enquiries

As with the Nichols case, enquiries would be made at local hospitals to trace any person who might have received treatment for injuries possibly sustained during the attack on Chapman.

7. Professional Informants

Local informants known to the police as being reliable would be requested to seek information that could assist the investigation.

8. Profiling

Profiles of the victim and her known associates or relatives would be completed. The Suspects or Offenders Profile in the Nichols case would be further developed.

9. Media

Public appeals for information and assistance would be made in the same way as in the first murder, and press conferences would be conducted in a similar fashion.

The following additional Lines of Enquiry would be given top priority during the initial stages of the investigation:

10. Envelope Recovered at the Scene
Efforts would be made to confirm whether the item had been in the victim's possession prior to the murder and, if so, from whom did she receive it? Those enquiries would be made whilst the part envelope was being forensically examined for fingerprints, fibres or other material or substance that could be present.

11. Leather Apron Found at Scene
Enquiries would be instigated to trace the owner of the article and eliminate the same from the investigation.

12. Property Recovered Near the Body
The brass rings, muslin and paper case would be submitted for fingerprint and forensic examination.

13. The Suspect William Henry Piggott
Further extensive enquiries by members of the investigation team would be made to eliminate Piggott from the investigation. Those enquiries could include the tracing of the woman he allegedly assaulted, possibly by using the media, and medical evidence to confirm the statement he had previously made.

The Senior Investigating Officer would then select his Management Team, each member having responsibility for managing individually defined Lines of Enquiry.

Annie May Chapman – Areas to be examined
Abberline would put the following questions to the Chapman Management Team:

1. Could the lack of blood found at the scene result from the majority being soaked up by the victim's clothing?

2. What was the exact time of death?

3. How could the victim have been subjected to such a violent attack and not have any clothing torn or ripped?

4. What similarities were there to the first murder?

5. Were there any witnesses who could have assisted with identifying the killer?

6. Were there any blood samples taken from the scene for comparison with the victim or suspect?

7. How would appeals for witnesses be used effectively?

8. What was the position of the first murder scene with that of the second murder?

9. How much consideration should be given to the killer wearing a disguise?

10. Could the money found on the body of the victim have been paid to her by the killer?

11. What enquiries could be made relative to the murder weapon?

1. Could the lack of blood found at the scene result from the majority being soaked up by the victim's clothing?
This would be a difficult question to answer today, and would certainly have been so one hundred years ago. Only close examination of the victim's clothing and a calculated guess would give the investigating officer any indication. In deciding whether or not the victim had been killed at the same location

where the body was found, signs of blood splashes in the immediate vicinity of the body would support a theory that the victim was attacked where the body was found. In the case of Annie Chapman, 'splashes of blood' were found on the fence near to where she lay, which would almost certainly prove that she was murdered there.

The scene would have been identified as including the front of the house, the passageway which led to the rear and the whole of the backyard in which the body was found. Any trace of blood at the front of the house or along the internal passageway would have been fundamental to the investigation. The possibility of the victim having been attacked away from where she was found would then have to be given serious consideration.

In circumstances where there was little blood found at the scene or in the body, then a wider search of the area would have to be carried out, with a view to identifying another scene. If those enquiries met with a negative result, then the location of the body would have to be treated as being the only scene.

2. *What was the exact time of death?*

If what the witness Cadosh stated was true, then death would have occurred at about 5.15 a.m. However, further information to corroborate that would be sought. It would appear that the victim was last seen alive by the landlord Timothy Donovan at 1.45 a.m. that morning. His testimony was supported by a nightwatchman, John Evans, who saw Chapman leave the lodging-house and walk towards Spitalfields Church. Therefore enquiries and appeals for help from the public would have to be made to try and establish Chapman's movements between 1.45 a.m. and 6.00 a.m., when she was found by the witness Davis.

Dr Phillips, who attended the scene and examined the body, thought that Annie Chapman had been dead for approximately

53

two hours before the time he commenced his examination at 6.30 a.m. This evidence conflicted with that given by the witness Cadosh; however, Dr Phillips did concede that the heavy loss of blood and the coldness of the early morning could have distorted his judgement.

3. How could the victim have been subjected to such a violent attack and not have any clothing torn or ripped?

The explanation is quite clear. For a number of reasons the victim might not have had the opportunity to resist her attacker. As with Mary Nichols, the post mortem revealed recent bruises on the face, particularly in the area of the chin. That would indicate that she was possibly throttled prior to her throat being cut, which would not give her the time or opportunity to try and fight off her attacker. Having disabled his victim, the killer could then mutilate other areas of the body without having to use force to remove clothing. On 26 September 1888, the coroner explained that the victim must have entered the yard willingly and in the company of her killer.

> '...they descended the three steps into the yard. The wretch must have then seized the deceased, perhaps with Judas-like approaches. He seized her by the chin. He pressed her throat, and while thus preventing the slightest cry, he at the same time produced insensibility and suffocation. There was no evidence of any struggle.'

Such a description of events most probably was an accurate one. Consideration would have to be given, however, to the victim's build. Annie Chapman was described by some of her friends as being a plump, well-proportioned woman. It could well be argued that such a woman would have managed to have put up a degree of resistance, unless of course there was

54

no warning of the attack. One other fact worthy of note was that she was suffering from tuberculosis at the time of her death, which could have resulted in her being much weaker than an average person of the same weight and proportion.

At the inquest, Phillips stated the following:

> '*The stomach contained a little food, but there was not any sign of fluid. There was no appearance of the deceased having taken alcohol, but there were signs of great deprivation ...*'

4. What similarities were there to the first murder?

As discussed previously, there were a number of linking factors that supported the theory that both women had been murdered by the same person. However, there would have to be sufficient evidence to support that claim before formally acknowledging that they were linked. The real difficulty exists for the Senior Investigating Officer when deciding how the linked enquiries should be structured and managed. Where investigations target a serial killer, then contingency plans must be made to deal with future crimes. If there is any doubt that a murder has been committed by a different person responsible for a number of crimes, then it should not be treated in isolation and become a part of the networked satellite system of Major Incident Rooms.

5. Were there any witnesses who could have assisted with identifying the killer?

Apart from the man Cadosh, the only witnesses were those who had seen Chapman some hours prior to her murder. At a time when early morning market workers were making their way to work in such a densely populated area, it is remarkable that no one saw anybody looking suspicious or hurrying away from the scene. A belief that the killer knew the area well and may have resided there, or was wearing clothing to naturally fit in with the neighbourhood, could have been a realistic one.

55

However, a senior investigating officer could be convinced that someone had seen the killer prior to or after the murder had been committed, although no witnesses had come forward. Members of the public needn't necessarily know that they have information valuable to the investigation, and it is the role of the police to ensure that everything is done to jog memories. Part of that process would be the reconstruction of each of the two murders, using the media to deliver messages to the public in the hope that there were positive responses.

6. Were there any blood samples taken from the scene for comparison with the victim or suspect?

At the time of the Whitechapel murders blood did not have the same significance in criminal investigation that it does today. With the introduction of DNA Profiling, blood, semen, hair and other human samples are important for the purposes of identifying individuals. At the scene of Annie Chapman's murder it would have been essential to have recovered what blood or other samples were available. Efforts would then have been made to match those samples belonging to the victim and identify other samples that were outstanding. The latter would most certainly have been used to forensically build a profile of the killer.

7. How would appeals for witnesses be used effectively?

In 1888 press circulations and distribution facilities were not as wide or effective as today. The media network consisted only of newspapers and journals, which usually contained illustrations or sketches made by freelance artists. Today both television and radio ensure that information is carried to the public with speed and effect. The relationships between the media and police have become more professional and senior investigating officers consider carefully the amount of information they are prepared to disclose during the early stages of an investigation. In time, the initial impact and public interest in a major criminal enquiry can dwindle, and it is possible to re-enforce awareness through subsequent press releases. In addition the quality of information released to support appeals for assistance from the public has increased in recent years.

8. What was the position of the first murder scene with that of the second murder?
The distance between the first two murders was less than half a mile. Such close proximity of the scenes would have been factors considered by the investigation team. Did the killer live in the Whitechapel area? Did he have relatives, friends or associates residing there? Was the killer employed in Whitechapel or connected with people living there? Was he a traveller who regularly passed through the neighbourhood? Lines of Enquiry should have been created and individuals falling within each of those parameters identified and investigated.

9. How much consideration should be given to the killer wearing a disguise?
Whitechapel would have been regularly visited by dockers and other characters attracted to the market area. Any person re-sembling a market worker or other occupation predominant in the area would not attract attention to themselves. However, during Victorian times, a person who was well dressed would be noticed but not challenged, because of the class distinctions that existed.

There could have been two reasons for the Ripper to have felt the need to disguise himself. Firstly, he could have lived in the Whitechapel area and was afraid of being recognized, or he could have belonged to a higher class of people than that residing in Whitechapel at that time and felt the need to wear clothing more appropriate to the area. One other consideration should have been given to the possibility of the murderer having employment that required the wearing of a uniform, such as police or armed forces.

10. Could the money found on the body of the victim have been paid to her by the killer?

That possibility is a real one, although forensic examination of the items today would not allow much room for optimism. If the denominations of the coins had been higher than what was usually possessed by a street prostitute, then suspicions that the killer could have come from a higher class of society would have been justified. If it was accepted that the payment had been made by the killer, then the *modus operandi* used would have included paying women prior to killing them, which would assist today in compiling a psychological profile. If, however, it was not suspected that any money had changed hands, then inferences could have been made that the victim had been with another client prior to meeting the killer. If that was the case, then appeals for help from the public to identify any person seeing the victim alive just prior to her death should have been made.

11. What enquiries could be made relative to the murder weapon?

Every effort should have been made to trace the weapon, which could have been discarded by the killer after the murder had been committed. Attempts should have been made to obtain a description of the weapon at the post mortem. The length and width of the blade could be ascertained together with other possible characteristics. A senior investigating officer should make sure that only facts from which a description is compiled are publicized and supposition ignored. Once satisfied that the description of the weapon is a fairly accurate one, that should be circulated as quickly and as widely as possible.

In addition, the information relevant to the type of weapon used should have been passed to the doctor who performed the post mortem for the first murder, and notes made by both pathologists should have been compared.

Three

A Revised Hypothesis

During the three-week period which followed the murder of Annie Chapman, Abberline had met daily with both senior investigating officers responsible for managing those investigations. On 22 September 1888, the Management Teams for both enquiries met, and Abberline asked for presentations to be made on the Lines of Enquiry and how they were progressing. He was informed of the following:

Nichols' clothing had been submitted to the Forensic Science Laboratory for detailed examination. A number of fibres recovered from her outer garments proved to be foreign to the articles of clothing she had been wearing at the time of her murder. Analysis of the fibres revealed that they were woollen and contained a black dye, the main component being a natural source of colouring obtained from blackberries, commonly grown in hedgerows in many European countries including Great Britain. Further enquiries were being made with clothing manufacturers and importers to trace tailors who supplied cloth containing similar dyed woollen fibres.

During the scene examination in Bucks Row a partial footprint impression was recovered from a patch of mud situated in the gutter near to where the body lay. The impression had been photographed before a plaster cast was made and sent to the Forensic Science Laboratory for further examination. The result received from the scientists revealed that the footprint had been made by a size 8 boot. The sole had ridges cut across the leather which were man-made and contained a number of characteristics which would only be applicable to the footwear that made the impression. Further enquiries had already revealed that it was common practice for seamen to cut ridges in the soles of their leather boots to obtain greater adhesion when on board ship. That information was being investigated further.

There was no further data available from the Nichols murder, and officers were continuing to investigate the identified Lines of Enquiry.

During the forensic examination of the Chapman murder scene, a number of fibres had been recovered from the wall immediately adjacent to the door leading to the rear yard of 29 Hanbury Street, and from an initial laboratory examination they appeared to resemble those fibres recovered from the Nichols scene.

In addition another footprint impression, similar to the one found at the Nichols scene, was discovered near the front door of number 29 Hanbury Street, again in a patch of dirt situated on the pavement. Together with the woollen fibres, a cast of the footprint had been submitted for forensic examination. The laboratory had not yet obtained any conclusive results, and scientists were continuing with their work.

In Old Montague Street, near to the Chapman murder scene, a police officer had recovered a bloodstained lady's handkerchief which was found lying discarded in the gutter. There had been confirmation from field tests that the item was stained with human blood, but further analysis and tests were required to establish whether or not the blood was that of the victim. The first tests, however, indicated that the blood was of a different group from that of Chapman.

When approached by police officers, Walter Graves remembered collecting a fare from St Katherine Docks at 12.15 a.m. on 8 September. The passenger was a man aged about 30 years, 5 feet 6 inches, slim build, with dark hair beneath a peaked ribbed cap and a black moustache waxed at both ends. Graves thought that the man had an accent but couldn't recognize whether it was English or foreign. The fare was dropped off at 12.25 a.m. in Aldgate at the junction with Commercial Street, only five minutes' walk from 29 Hanbury Street. Graves had made a full witness statement.

During the enquiries made with members of the medical profession, a number of surgeons had been interviewed in local hospitals, and although some diverse opinions had been obtained as to whether or not the killer would have had some anatomical knowledge, no real progress had been made. These enquiries were proving to be extremely difficult because of the high level of respect police officers in general held for members of the medical profession. Abberline directed that he wanted all information and opinions passed to his officers by those interviewed, challenged and probed.

Enquiries made at the London hospitals failed to trace any person who possibly required treatment to injuries sustained during the attacks on Chapman and Nichols. Throughout central London a total number of 12 patients had been missing from various mental institutions on the dates of the murders, but they had all been eventually accounted for and eliminated from the investigations.

A number of descriptive points taken from witness statements had been compiled and released to the press. A Psychological Profile was being developed further as additional information was being obtained and inputted into the Major Incident Room computer database.

The Crime Pattern Analysis study had found no evidence to support a theory that the 'Ripper' could have been committing other crimes apart from the murders. Abberline was satisfied that, whatever the motive behind the killings, he was searching for an homicidal maniac who needed to be caught as quickly as possible, rather than a burglar or other type of criminal.

Following the briefing on 22 September 1888, Abberline instructed selected groups of detectives to concentrate on three major areas: the shoe description, the dyed woollen fibres, and the description of the assailant that was now becoming fairly detailed. He also directed that a number of detectives be given the responsibility of tracing the fare taken to Whitechapel by the witness Graves.

One national newspaper had already published its own version of an artist's sketch of what the murderer looked like. That put further pressure on Abberline to release an official police sketch as soon as possible. Based on the information provided by Graves, the following sketch was given to the press together with a statement placing some emphasis on the 'waxed moustache'. The press release also requested any person who may have known the identity of a man with a similar description, who had visited Whitechapel on the night of Annie Chapman's murder, to come forward.

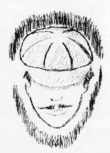

The media can pressure the police into releasing an artist's impression, no matter how little information is available at the time.

Abberline confirmed that the remaining Lines of Enquiry would continue, with the exception of the Crime Pattern Analysis, which would cease forthwith.

At this stage of the investigations Abberline was fairly satisfied that enquiries were being completed expeditiously and some progress was being made. He was also optimistic that the murderer would be caught, but there was much more work to be done.

On 25 September 1888, the following letter was received by Detective Superintendent Abberline at Scotland Yard:

Dear Detective Superintendent Abberline,
I am a Bachelor of Science and Master of Science and I have been a forensic scientist for twenty years.

I have dealt with numerous cases involving the examination of items similar to those that are subject of this report.

On Friday, 31 August 1888, Detective Constable Burt brought to the laboratory two items marked SB 1 and SB 2. Both were contained in sealed plastic bags and were labelled as exhibits. I took possession of both items and found them to be securely packaged and adequately labelled.

I was informed that the items had been recovered from the murder scene of Mary Ann Nichols in Bucks Row, Whitechapel, on Friday, 31 August 1888.

ITEM SB1
This exhibit consisted of six strands of fibre of varying lengths.
ITEM SB2
This exhibit consisted of a plaster cast of a footprint impression.
INFORMATION RE ITEM SB1
Purpose of Examination
To try and identify the material of each fibre strand and any other substance present.
Results of Examination
Each fibre strand was made of natural wool and contained a quantity of blackberry juice. On further analysis of the fluid taken from the fibres no other component was identifiable. In my opinion, the blackberry juice had been used as a form of dye.

INFORMATION RE ITEM SB2

Purpose of Examination

To identify the type of footwear responsible for the print and isolate any characteristics belonging to that footwear.

Result of Examination

The impression was made by a size 8 heavy boot which originally had a plain sole.

From my own sketch of the indentation marks illustrated below, the patterns at A and B are not machine-made. The inconsistencies that exist within the patterns show that deeper cuts had been made on the outside of the sole. This is consistent with greater pressure being applied to a sharp instrument at the beginning of each cut and lesser as the instrument is moved across the sole. In my opinion the cuts were made deliberately and by hand.

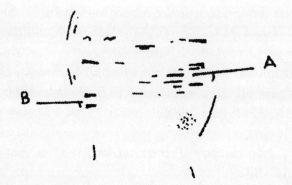

Exhibit No. WB1

There are a number of similar items recovered from the scene of the murder of Annie May Chapman in Hanbury Street on 8 September 1888. These will be subject of further reports and statements.

Yours sincerely,

(signed) W Bliss

B.Sc. M.Sc.

Four

Double Murder

ELIZABETH STRIDE

'There were no mutilations similar to the previous two murders'

A tidal wave of fear swept through London's East End following the murders of Mary Ann Nichols and Annie May Chapman. Horror stories of how the killer had chosen his victims and what he had done with them became exaggerated. Descriptions of a monster looking for women and children to slay, and later eat, became abundant in local public houses and other meeting places. People found a common interest that was now the most important issue in their lives. Newspapers and journals fuelled the anxiety with inaccurate reports and false allegations that added to the difficulties the police were experiencing from the growing pressure demanding the killer's capture. Various communal groups living and working in Whitechapel became more closely bonded, and people turned to each other for support and comfort.

In 1888 the majority of news travelled by way of verbal communication, and residents took advantage of every opportunity to meet together. Public houses saw a rapid increase in trade. People met on street corners to discuss what they had heard about the murders and the investigations that were taking place. Individuals became locked in their own ideas and thoughts about the kind of man the police were looking for. A general picture of a 'bogey man' who would kill more women if not caught quickly soon emerged and spread quickly throughout London. The hardships that usually accompanied poverty were temporarily forgotten and the population became totally gripped by the man who was already referred to as 'Jack the Ripper'.

Detective Inspector Abberline soon found himself the subject of criticism by senior officers at Scotland Yard, demanding a quick result to the high-profile investigation. He initially concentrated his enquiries on the two murder scenes, and numerous suspects were arrested and interviewed, but were later released by Abberline's officers. Failure to secure an early result soon led to the police becoming the target of dissatisfaction and criticism. Sir Charles Warren, the metropolitan commissioner of police, became aware of the increasing criticism and public concern about himself and his officers. A number of Vigilance Committees were formed to try and prevent further murders being committed. Some members included people with good intentions, but more politically motivated individuals were also ever-present, leading the street meetings that took place. Public subscriptions were collected and rewards offered for information that would lead to the Ripper's identity, but there was no untoward incident for a three-week period that followed the discovery of Annie Chapman's body.

During the early hours of Sunday, 30 September, two episodes occurred in the Ripper series, which left the population of London in a state of outrage. Louis Diemschutz lived with his wife at a Working Men's Club in Berner Street, Whitechapel. At night, he and his wife were employed there as the steward and stewardess. During the daytime, Diemschutz worked on a stall in a nearby open market selling cheap jewellery. On Saturday, 29 September, he spent the day at Westow Hill Market, Sydenham, trying to make enough money to tide him over for the remainder of the weekend. At the end of the day he made his way home with his horse and cart and, as was his habit, decided to stop for a beverage at the Grove Tavern situated in Lordship Lane. Diemschutz then continued on his homeward journey. At 12.55 a.m. he turned into Berner Street and thought it best to leave some of the unsold goods with his wife, before stabling the horse in a nearby yard.

The Working Men's Club was situated on one side of a narrow court in Berner Street. The entrance to it was through a pair of large wooden gates. Opposite the club there were several mean houses, mostly occupied by Polish and German Jews. The yard gates were open, and Diemschutz could see through them what appeared to be a bundle of clothes lying on the floor. He poked the clothing with his whip, but there was no movement or sound. He could see that it was a woman, but thought that she was in a drunken sleep.

The night was damp and miserable, and Diemschutz saw that there were still people at the club before he made his way inside and was greeted by his wife. The steward's first priority was to return outside to the open yard and deal with the 'drunken woman' lying on the floor. He lit a candle and returned to awaken and eject the motionless wretch from the property.

As Diemschutz walked across the dimly lit yard he could hear the voices coming from inside the club, but for some unknown reason, felt a little nervous as he approached the bundle of clothing. He felt that something was wrong; there appeared to be an eerie atmosphere which made him feel cold and shaky. Diemschutz stopped just short of where the woman lay and looked back towards the lights shining through the windows of the club; they offered him some comfort. He then turned and looked hard into the four dark corners of the yard but couldn't see anyone or anything. His hands started to shake, but he didn't know why. He felt that 'the eyes of evil were watching me from the darkness'. He called out to the motionless woman lying there, but didn't hear any reply. As he raised the candle higher to obtain more light, he looked down and gazed into the tortured face of the female. He looked closer and saw that her throat had been cut, exposing a severe gash that had completely severed the windpipe and left carotid artery. It was a gruesome sight and Diemschutz's fear was replaced by terror as he dropped the candle onto the cobbled stones and screamed for help. The horrified steward was soon joined by others from the club.

The victim's left arm was bent above her head whilst her right arm rested against an old grating. Her legs were drawn up, and in her right hand she was still clutching a small packet of pink cachous, used to sweeten the breath. In her left hand she held what appeared to be several grapes. The body of the woman was later identified to be that of a known local prostitute. The third victim of the Ripper.

Elizabeth Stride had been born near Gothenburg in Sweden in 1843. She came to London in 1866, and during the early years of her marriage to a carpenter by the name of Thomas Stride she helped raise three children. It is believed that both Elizabeth and Thomas managed a coffee-house in London's East End until, it was alleged at the time, a boating tragedy on the River Thames resulted in the deaths of her husband and children. There is, however, no evidence to substantiate that claim, and in the early part of 1888 Elizabeth Stride met a man named Michael Kidney, who she was living with at the time of her murder. Their stormy relationship had lasted for approximately three years. According to Kidney, Stride would disappear for a number of days following violent arguments between them.

William West had been visiting the club on the night of the murder, and at 12.30 a.m. had gone outside into the yard to escape the smoky atmosphere and enjoy a breath of fresh air. He was adamant that the body of Stride was not there at that particular time. That information led the police to believe that the prostitute had been murdered between West's visit to the yard at 12.30 a.m. and 12.55 a.m., when Diemschutz first arrived on the scene and saw what he then thought was a drunk lying on the floor.

Doctor Frederick Blackwell later confirmed that, apart from the cut throat, there were no other marks on the body. There were no mutilations similar to the previous two murders. However, it was accepted at the time that the killer could have been disturbed by the arrival of Diemschutz. That could explain why, whilst the police and doctors were examining the body of Elizabeth Stride, another prostitute killing took place nearby.

CATHARINE EDDOWES

'The face had been disfigured by knife slashes, both eyes had been injured and part of the right ear was missing'

Those police officers examining the scene in Berner Street were not aware at the time that another prostitute was being brutally murdered, only a few hundred yards away. In fact Mitre Square was less than ten minutes' walking distance along Commercial Road, Aldgate, and into Mitre Street. It was also a section of Police Constable Watkins' beat, and at 1.30 a.m. on Sunday, 30 September 1888, the patrolling officer walked into the Square to examine the security of doors, windows and padlocks. His presence would have been noticed by the light flashing from his 'Bullseye' lantern. Everything at that time appeared to be in order, so the officer continued on his way.

Approximately 15 minutes later PC Watkins returned to Mitre Square to repeat his examination of that part of his beat. Upon reaching the south-west corner of the square, his lantern lit up an object lying on the floor. It was the body of a woman staring up at him from the darkness of the street cobbles upon which she lay. There was a look of intense horror on the dead woman's face. The officer was startled and could only stare back into the woman's eyes as he felt his knees start to tremble. He tried to speak to her, although he knew she was dead, but his throat and mouth were dry and incapable of putting words together. He wanted to turn around and look about him, but couldn't. The police officer felt paralysed by the shock of walking into such an alarming and terrifying sight. He stood motionless for a short while, trying to decide what to do. After what appeared to have been an eternity, calmness and normality started to return. The police officer remembered the nightwatchman who was employed in a warehouse just down the street, and ran to get his assistance.

The wounds and mutilations to the body of Catharine Eddowes were considerable. The throat was cut, the abdomen mutilated and some of the internal organs removed. PC Watkins later told the inquest that the body was lying on its back and had been 'ripped up like a pig in the market…there was a big gash up the stomach, the entrails were torn out and flung in a heap about her neck'.

Both Watkins and Herbert Morris, the nightwatchman, gave evidence at the inquest that assisted in identifying the time Eddowes had met her death. Morris stated that he had not heard any sounds in the square that night except the footsteps of PC Watkins when patrolling on the first occasion. The police officer swore that the body had not been there when he patrolled Mitre Square 15 minutes before finding the dead woman.

Catharine Eddowes was born in Wolverhampton and was 46 years of age at the time of her murder. Her family had moved to Bermondsey in London before she was two, and her mother died just after the young Catharine had reached her thirteenth birthday. Following a period in a workhouse and industrial school, she returned to the Wolverhampton area, where it is alleged she married a local man, Thomas Conway. They lived together for almost 20 years during which time there were three children, two sons and a daughter. There is little doubt that Eddowes experienced most of the hardships of life in Victorian England during her early years, and following her separation from Conway in 1880, moved back down to London, where she lived with John Kelly, initially in Flower and Dean Street, Whitechapel.

Eddowes and Kelly remained together for approximately seven years, until her death. She was often in the habit of pawning property or trying other means to scrape together sufficient money for a meal or drink, and would use Kelly's name as well as many others. During the time they were together, they lived mostly in common lodging-houses in the Thrawl Street area of Whitechapel, and Catharine was known to sell trinkets on the streets during the daytime, working as a common prostitute at night. Her common-law husband was an unemployed casual labourer who had not experienced much luck or good fortune during his lifetime. They lived mostly in a state of destitution, and even on the day before she met her death, Catharine had pawned John Kelly's shirt and boots to get enough money to buy food.

At 8.30 p.m. on the night of her murder, PCs Robinson and Simmons arrested Eddowes for being drunk and disorderly in Aldgate High Street, after finding her lying in the gutter, causing a disturbance. She was taken to Bishopsgate Police Station, where she remained in a cell until being released at about 1.00 a.m. She had given her name and address as being Mary Ann Kelly of 6 Fashion Street. Her last recorded words upon being released were 'Good night, old cock'.

Mitre Square was only a few minutes' walk from Bishopsgate Police Station, and it was assumed at the time that Eddowes had walked directly there after being given her

73

freedom back. She was wearing a black straw bonnet trimmed with green and black velvet and black beads, a black cloth jacket with imitation fur edging around the collar and sleeves, and a flower-patterned skirt with an apron that had once been white in colour, but was now almost black from dirt and grime.

Within an hour of the discovery of the fourth Ripper victim, Police Constable Alfred Long came across a piece of blood-stained apron in a building in Goulston Street, which again wasn't very far away from the murder scene. The bloodstained cloth, found in a dark passageway leading to some flats, fitted exactly with a piece missing from the apron worn by Eddowes. The following message was written in chalk on a blackened wall, above where the piece of cloth had been found:

*'The Juwes are The men That Will
not be Blamed for nothing.'*

That same night, the Police Commissioner, Sir Charles Warren, visited the scenes of both murders and allegedly ordered the writing on the wall to be removed. It is believed that the reason why Warren made that decision was because he thought the words could aggravate prejudices against the local Jewish community, which could have resulted in public disorders between rival groups. His orders were reluctantly carried out.

Following the discovery of the bloodstained piece of apron, detectives visited nearby Dorset Street, which was north of Goulston Street and adjacent to Crispin Street. There, in a public wash-basin, they found what they believed to be blood-stains. It was thought at the time that the murderer had possibly stopped in Dorset Street to wash his hands before continuing along his escape route.

The murders of Stride and Eddowes represented the worst possible situation for both the police and government officials. Fears grew within the corridors of power that the murders could lead to outbreaks of public disorder because Whitechapel was no longer safe for women to walk the streets. The killer had to be caught before any further atrocities were committed. There were strong words spoken in all quarters, and feelings of anger both towards the killer and the police, for what was seen as their failures, swelled throughout the capital.

Stride and Eddowes – An Hypothesis, One Hundred Years On

Detective Superintendent Abberline returned to his office at Scotland Yard having visited both the Stride and Eddowes murder scenes. He knew that the time was approaching when the investigations would be reviewed by another senior investigating officer. This is common practice in circumstances where a murder has not been detected within a 28-day period and Abberline welcomed the opportunity to obtain the objective views of another senior colleague. However, for the time being he was in need of solitude, and for a while sat alone in the safe environment of his office.

The senior detective leaned backwards in his chair and staring up at the ceiling, locked within his own thoughts and ideas. His mind started to race from one synopsis to another until it became flooded with confusion. He drank numerous cups of tea until he thought it was bellowing out of his ears, and smoked cigars which turned his office into a fog. Eventually Abberline began to focus more easily upon the structural side of the investigations. He tried to devise what he thought would be the most efficient and effective way to progress the enquiries, knowing that strong leadership would now be required to maintain the team spirit that had developed during the past four weeks amongst his officers and staff.

There were a number of issues that were still ambiguous and caused Abberline some concern. If the killer lived locally, then why hadn't there been any information coming off the streets that could help to identify him? Abberline was convinced that no one would deliberately shelter a man responsible for crimes of this nature. If he wasn't a local man, then how did he travel into Whitechapel and then leave without being seen? Did he walk, which was doubtful, or travel by carriage? Did he have an accomplice? If so, then the accomplice must have played a minor role, for this was the work of one man. That being the case, then following the publicity the murders had attracted, it was surprising the accomplice hadn't come forward with the killer's identity.

Abberline had a wealth of experience in dealing with major criminal investigations, and questioned his own actions to try and identify something he might have overlooked. His thought patterns were interrupted by the telephone ringing. It was Abberline's commanding officer, Detective Chief Super-intendent Arnold.

'Fred, the Commissioner has asked me to do the Review personally, starting this morning. He wants a report from me within the week.'

Abberline felt completely drained from the events of the previous few weeks, but was ready to assist Arnold in any way he could. He agreed to meet the Detective Chief Superintendent later that day at Scotland Yard. He would allow the Reviewing Officer access to his operational plans and strategies, including his Policy File, which had been maintained throughout the murder enquiries and was a complete record of every policy decision Abberline had made, together with the reasons for making those decisions.

Following a short conversation with Arnold, Abberline sat back and returned to his personal thoughts on how the investigations were now to be progressed. He was soon overcome by sleep and later awakened, more refreshed and ready to throw himself back into the mainstream investigative work, once he had stimulated himself further with a cup of coffee.

Post Mortem on Stride

Doctors Blackwell and Phillips performed the post mortem on Elizabeth Stride. When examining the body, they found bruising on both shoulders and chest, but there were no facial contusions present. The victim's clothing had not been disturbed, although a silk scarf wrapped around her neck had been frayed by the knife used to cut her throat. That was the only incision found on the body and began on the left side, $2^1/_2$ inches below the angle of the jaw. The windpipe had been cut through, although none of the blood vessels in the neck had been severed. Such findings would have indicated that the knife used was partially blunt, unlike the weapon involved in the previous two murders. However, both doctors believed that the knife used would have been a sharp pointed instrument.

Post Mortem on Eddowes

Doctor Phillips also attended the post mortem on Catharine Eddowes, together with Doctors Brown, Sequierra and Saunders. The walls to the abdomen had been laid open and the left kidney and uterus had been removed. There was also disfigurement to the face: both eyes had been damaged by knife slashes and part of the victim's right ear was missing. The throat had been cut wide open, and the weapon used was believed to have been a knife with a long narrow-pointed blade.

Following the post mortems on Stride and Eddowes, Abberline called a meeting of his senior detectives at Scotland Yard. There they also met Arnold and his Review Team. The Chief Superintendent had appointed a detective inspector to examine the database supporting the investigations. That officer's job would be to ensure that policies were being adhered to. He also tasked a finance officer with analysing the budgetary issues involved and presenting him with a financial projection outlining future costs and expenses. The third member of Arnold's team was a detective sergeant who would be responsible for looking at the welfare issues relevant to police officers and support staff. Arnold himself would examine the Senior Investigating Officers' Policy Files, including Abberline's, and discuss any recognized issues with individual officers.

The murders of Stride and Eddowes were discussed in depth prior to Arnold commencing his Review, and the following factors were outlined:

1. As with the previous two murders, both victims were common prostitutes.

2. The killer had used a pointed knife with a long, narrow blade in both attacks, according to the pathologists.

3. The attacks took place in the Whitechapel area.

4. The killer committed his crimes during the hours of darkness with the knowledge that police officers and members of the public were aware of his threat and street patrols had been increased.

5. Stride was subjected to a lesser degree of violence than Eddowes, which supported the theory that the killer had been disturbed by the witness Diemschutz.

6. The Eddowes murder was committed without noticeable noise from the victim or killer, if the presence of the night-watchman and patrolling police officer are believed.

7. The severity of the violence to which Eddowes had been subjected was more intense than that used against the other victims, which could have been the result of the killer's frustration becoming more extreme.

8. There was still no apparent motive.

9. The movements of the killer between the scenes of the first and second murders support the belief that his knowledge of the area was a detailed one, although Abberline doubted that he resided locally.

10. The information obtained from the first two Ripper murders confirmed that the killer retained possession of the murder weapon after each crime.

Abberline decided that the Lines of Enquiry for the Stride and Eddowes murders would be the same as those identified in the previous two cases, with three additions.

1. The writing on the wall
The message, 'The Juwes are The men That Will not be Blamed for nothing', meant nothing, and there was no logical reason why the murderer would have written it, except to draw attention to the piece of apron found on the floor. However, enquiries would concentrate on two aspects: firstly, the hand-

writing, which would be submitted for expert analysis, hopefully to obtain as much information as possible about the author. Secondly, professional assistance would be sought to decipher any hidden message that might be contained within the words written. There could have been a possibility that the words were in fact coded, although doubtful. Abberline would want to try and clarify whether or not the message represented anything of significance and whether it could be connected to the killer.

2. The bloodstained apron
This would be regarded as a vital clue concerning the character of the murderer and his escape route from the scene of the Eddowes murder. The first question would be to ask why the killer went to the trouble of removing the segment from the victim's apron? Why would he then carry it away from the scene, only to discard it a few streets away? A possible answer would be that the Ripper intended to take away with him a momento of his latest murder. If that was the case, then if the cloth had been found in the street it might have been easier to accept that it had been dropped accidentally by the killer as he fled away from Mitre Square. However, it had been found in an enclosed passageway. This could indicate that the item had been discarded deliberately, either because the Ripper no longer wished to retain it, and if so, why? Or he had left it in anticipation that it would be found. If that was the case, then he wished to let the police know the escape route he had decided to take. If that was so, then either he had a desire to be caught or his unstable and twisted mind was regarding the past efforts and failures of the police to catch him, with contempt.

The bloodstained apron would be submitted for forensic examination to confirm that the blood came from the victim and to trace any other fibres or material present on the cloth.

3. The bloodstains in the public wash-basin

Field tests would have already confirmed to Abberline that the stains were human blood. Forensic scientists would then be requested to recover samples for laboratory analysis, to confirm whether or not the blood came from either of the victims. A DNA Profile would also be completed if the samples did not belong to Catharine Eddowes or Elizabeth Stride.

Elizabeth Stride and Catharine Eddowes – Areas to be examined

Abberline and his Management Team discussed the following questions:

1. Was it right to link both the Stride and Eddowes murders?

2. Was there sufficient evidence available to link Stride and Eddowes with the murders of Nichols and Chapman?

3. Could the Stride and Eddowes murder scenes have been visited by the same person in the time allowed to travel the distance that separated them?

4. How could the murderer have enjoyed such freedom of movement between both crime scenes without being detected?

5. Why were there no mutilations on Stride's body?

6. How could the murder of Catharine Eddowes have been committed without the nightwatchman working in Mitre Square hearing or seeing anything?

7. Why did the Commissioner of Police order the writing on the wall to be cleaned off, leaving no trace?

8. When Eddowes was released from Bishopsgate Police Station, why was she not followed by police officers, taking into account the previous murders that had been committed in that area?

9. Was there any motive established at this stage?

10. Were there any signs of the killer wishing to communicate with the investigating officers?

11. What would be the major Lines of Enquiry today?

1. Was it right to link both the Stride and Eddowes murders? It would be difficult not to accept that the two murders were committed by the same person, although today comparisons would be charted and positive links identified. The following facts would support a linked enquiry:

1. The close proximity of the two murder scenes.

2. The antecedents of the victims and their trades, i.e. both common prostitutes.

3. The times that both crimes were committed, within minutes of each other.

4. The degrees of violence used against the victims.

5. The type of murder weapon used on each occasion, although there was some doubt as to whether or not the

same instrument had been used in both murders. There were signs that the knife used against Stride was blunt.

6. The positions of the bodies, i.e. both left in public places in similar postures.

7. The lack of a positive motive being identified from both cases.

8. Existing knowledge that the two previous murders of Nichols and Chapman were committed in the same area.

9. Each victim had her throat cut.

Consideration would be given today to the possibility of copycat crimes, but would be negated by the amount of violence and *modus operandi* or methods used by the killer. However, the possibility would still exist that Stride was the victim of a domestic murder, and the fact that it occurred on the same night as another Ripper murder could have been coincidental.

2. What was the evidence available to link the murders of Stride and Eddowes with the previous two Ripper killings?
The linking factors have been identified in the answer to question 1. The methods used by the killer would be important, such as the fact that the four victims were killed before mutilations took place. Evidentially, without having possession of the weapon used to murder Eddowes, it would have been difficult for the police to prove that the same person murdered Stride. What should be considered at this stage is the possibility of the killer having visited Whitechapel before the first murder. Public appeals for help should now have been accompanied by press releases drawing the public's attention to any suspected

person having been seen in the area before Nichols was murdered.

The linking of the four murders would create a pool of information collected from each of the investigations. The Intelligence Analyst would be given the job of extracting whatever common factors were present in each of the murders. Sequence of Events Charts would be compiled and profiles of each of the victims developed and examined for any common features.

A Psychological Profile of the murderer would attempt to identify the mental characteristics of the person responsible. Important factors, such as the period of time that elapsed between the first two murders and those of Stride and Eddowes, together with the increased level of violence used on Eddowes, would assist in compiling such a profile of the killer.

3. Could the Stride and Eddowes murder scenes have been visited by the same person in the time allowed to travel the distance that separated them?

It could be assumed that the murder of Elizabeth Stride occurred between 12.50 a.m. and 12.55 a.m., when the witness Diemschutz came onto the scene and obviously prevented the killer from completing his work. The second murder was discovered at approximately 1.45 a.m., which meant that Catharine Eddowes could have been fatally attacked sometime between 1.25 a.m. and 1.35 a.m. The average person walks approximately three miles in one hour. The distance between Berner Street and Mitre Square was about 1,150 yards which would have taken the killer approximately 15 minutes to have walked. Those time parameters would have left the murderer with at least 15 minutes to spare.

The distance between Mitre Square and Goulston Street was approximately 600 yards which would have taken between seven and ten minutes to walk. The killer would have arrived in Goulston Street, where the bloodstained apron was found, at approximately 1.45 a.m.

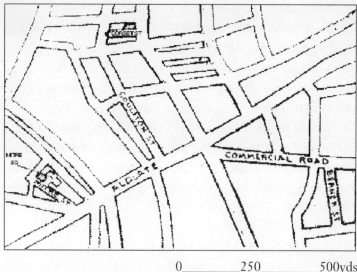

0_____250_____500yds

Street Map showing Berner Street, Mitre Square, Goulston Street and Dorset Street, Whitechapel.

4. How could the murderer have enjoyed such freedom of movement between both crime scenes without being detected? This is one question which will probably never be answered conclusively. There have been a number of other murder investigations where the police have failed to trace eyewitnesses who saw the killer. In reality, an individual responsible for committing a crime could have been seen by a large number of persons, but unless those potential witnesses are aware of the importance of what they have seen, it appears to them at the time to be insignificant. In circumstances where the mind fails to retain specific information, the police have been known to try a number of methods in an attempt to jog the memory. Cognitive interviewing is a technique used to recall in a witness' mind what was actually seen or heard, by attempting to trigger the subconscious into throwing forward a more detailed picture than what the witness has described. There have been occasions when witnesses have been subjected to professional hypnosis and a degree of success has been achieved.

Details of street patrols not deployed by the police in the Whitechapel area on 30 September are not available, but today any person known to have been present in the areas of Berner Street and Mitre Square at the appropriate times would be interviewed to solicit what information they had. Criticism must also be made of the Bishopsgate Police, who failed to provide protection for Catharine Eddowes. She was known to them as a prostitute and was allowed to leave police custody late at night, to walk in an area in which two murders of prostitutes had previously been committed.

A witness, William Marshall, who lived in Berner Street, told police officers that at about 11.45 p.m. that night he had seen Elizabeth Stride talking to a man in Berner Street. He described the man as being middle-aged, plump build, about 5 feet 6 inches tall, wearing a black coat and dark trousers. He also had a round peaked cap on his head and gave the appearance of being a clerk. The man was overheard to say to Stride, '*You could say anything but your prayers.*'

Police Constable William Smith saw a man of a similar description given by Marshall and a woman standing together at about 12.30 a.m. in Berner Street. The officer's story was supported by another witness, James Brown, who was working in a chandlers' shop in Berner Street and stated that he saw the same man and woman at about the same time as did PC Smith. As a result, the descriptions given by Smith and Brown were published in the *Police Gazette*:

At 12.35 a.m. 30th September, with Elizabeth Stride found murdered on the same date in Berner Street at 1 a.m., a man, age 28, height 5 feet 8 inches, complexion dark, small dark

moustache; dress, black diagonal coat, hard felt hat, collar and tie,
respectable appearance, carried a parcel wrapped up in newspaper.
At 12.45 a.m., 30th, with the same woman in Berner Street,
a man, age about 30, height 5 feet 5 inches; complexion fair,
hair dark, small brown moustache, full face, broad shoulders;
dress, dark jacket and trousers, black cap with peak.

Today the witnesses would have been asked to assist with a computer composite of the man's face, followed by an artist's impression. That information would be circulated nationally, with a request for the person involved to come forward for elimination purposes. There is little doubt that the witnesses saw the face of Jack the Ripper, although there was some confusion about actual times. Whether or not the 'newspaper package' contained the murder weapon will never be known. However, initial enquiries made at both murder scenes would have been aimed towards recovering bloodstained newspaper.

5. Why were there no mutilations on Stride's body?

Consideration should have been given to this question when deciding whether or not both murders had been committed by the same person. Some regard should have been given to the fact that the level of violence used against Stride was far less than that used against the other victims. There is little doubt that if Diemschutz had arrived in Berner Street minutes, or perhaps even seconds, before he actually did, he would have come face to face with the killer. There is also the possibility that the murderer remained at the scene and watched Diemschutz's actions before the steward entered the Working Men's Club. It does appear obvious that the killer was interrupted before he could complete his vile work.

Because of the strong possibility that the Ripper could still have been present on the scene when Diemschutz arrived back at the club, the witness would be subjected to cognitive interviewing. Professional hypnosis could also be considered to ascertain whether or not the steward actually saw or heard the murderer.

6. How could the murder of Catharine Eddowes have been committed without the nightwatchman working in Mitre Square hearing or seeing anything?

The witness Morris would have been subjected to the same interviewing processes as suggested for Diemschutz. Investigating officers are often frustrated by the lack of information obtained from potential witnesses, knowing that they should have seen or heard more than what they are saying. It is also easy to be wise after the event, and it must be accepted that ordinary members of the public go about their business not looking for things which a trained eye would more easily see.

7. Why did the Commissioner of Police order the writing on the wall to be cleaned off leaving no trace?

Such action was without doubt a mistake. It was criticized at the time, and would most certainly have been condemned in a major investigation today. The handwriting should have been photographed so that later comparisons could have been made with samples taken from suspects. A lot of positive information can be obtained from expert examination of handwriting samples, such as a person's character and whether or not the author was male or female, right- or left-handed, which would certainly have been beneficial to the Ripper enquiries bearing in mind the opinion of Dr Llewellyn in the Nichols murder, that the killer was left-handed. Also the immediate area surrounding the writing on the wall and where the piece of bloodstained apron had been found would now be forensically examined. Requests would be made to identify the material used to write the message and to recover any fibres or other material that could have been left by the killer.

The Commissioner was concerned that local residents and early morning workers would see the writing and interpret the message in such a way that verbal and physical attacks would be made upon members of the Jewish community. His greatest worry was that communal feelings could then become a flashpoint for organized public disorders and perhaps even riots. It is suggested that public appeals could have been made for any person having knowledge of the writing, without disclosing the contents, to come forward. There were no witnesses to the writing, but if it had been confirmed that the message was written before the bloodstained apron had been dropped, then the two incidents could have been isolated from each other. If it was accepted that the same person was responsible for both incidents, then the handwriting on the wall could have become an essential part of the investigation and subjected to further enquiries. If that was the case, then a number of options could have been considered by the Senior Investigating Officer. Either the murderer was becoming careless, or he deliberately left clues behind him to torment or communicate with those investigating his crimes.

8. When Eddowes was released from Bishopsgate Police Station, why was she not followed by police officers, taking into account the previous murders that had been committed in that area?
This was a careless mistake by the Bishopsgate Police, which cost Eddowes her life and perhaps lost an opportunity to capture the killer. If the victim had been followed, her life could have been spared and the murderer caught. One other aspect is that the fifth Ripper murder would not have occurred if the serial killer had been incarcerated. The reasons for not showing such initiative probably resulted from a lack of thought and incompetence, or a shortage of available police officers to carry out such an operation at that time. The first

explanation seems to be a more logical one and is more acceptable.

9. Was there any motive established at this stage?

The most difficult murders to detect are those that have no apparent motive. A senior investigating officer needs to identify a motive from which he can direct the Lines of Enquiry necessary to bring about a successful conclusion. Whether a crime is committed for sexual reasons, theft or revenge, the axis upon which most major investigations revolve is strongly dependent upon that knowledge. There was no motive identified in any of the Ripper murders, which meant that the investigations could not be restricted to narrow and specific Lines of Enquiry. The police officers engaged on the investigation would have been tasked with enquiries that were wide and far reaching. The tighter and more compact an investigation, the easier it is to manage which naturally promotes greater efficiency.

A popular theory put forward by individual researchers and criminologists during the past one hundred years or so, is that the killer had a grudge against one individual woman who was a common prostitute and worked in the Whitechapel area of London. It has been suggested that his search for that person resulted in five women being murdered. However, what is factual is that the intentions and desires of this particular serial killer went beyond the understanding and acceptability of human behaviour, both in 1888 and now. What is surprising is that, having achieved success by committing so many murders without detection, the killer kept returning to the same locality, obviously with the knowledge that the public in that district would be extremely vigilant and searching for him.

10. Were there any signs of the killer wishing to communicate with the investigating officers?

There have been a number of occasions throughout history when a person responsible for committing a serious crime has deliberately left clues or signs which have led to their arrest and later conviction. A common practice for some murderers is to take a 'souvenir' or 'reminder' of what they have accomplished: a piece of the victim's clothing or other item. A number have written to senior investigating officers, boasting of their success and challenging the police to catch them. In the Ripper cases the finding of the piece of bloodstained apron is very significant. The killer could have taken the article intending to keep the same as a momento, but later dropped it in Goulston Street by accident. It is suggested that such an act is highly unlikely because of where the item was found, as discussed earlier.

Another explanation is that the piece of apron could have been left deliberately to attract attention to the message on the wall, or to the direction he was travelling when escaping from the scene. In either case, it could have been recognized as a means of communication with the police. If that was so, then the killer's mental state and thought patterns were changing. It is suggested that the failure to secure his capture was resulting in an increase in the killer's levels of confidence. Such actions could have been interpreted as a way of showing contempt towards his pursuers or, more likely, giving them a red herring which could lead them away from the real escape route.

Another reason could be the possibility that the killer was making a cry for help. If the Ripper was suffering from a form of schizophrenia and there existed an element of conflict in his mental state – one part of his mind urging him to continue his horrific deeds and another telling him to stop – then a desire to communicate could be present. Perhaps his actions in Goulston Street could have been interpreted as being those initial signs of a wish to receive help? If the Senior Investigating Officer recognized the feasibility of the murderer wishing to communicate with him, he should also accept the possibility that such actions would be repeated in the future, either in writing or by some other means.

11. *What would be the Major Lines of Enquiry today?*
The Lines of Enquiry in a major investigation are essential to give it both management and operational direction. Where there is a need to solve problems or achieve objectives, there should be a strategic plan aimed towards supporting the methods in which those goals are to be reached. Greater emphasis is placed on planning and strategic analysis by senior investigating officers today, than ever before. When a major investigation is at 'A' and needs to go to the objective set at 'B', the Lines of Enquiry should direct the way in which the investigation is going to travel in order to reach 'B'. Careful consideration should be given by the Senior Investigating Officer to all the facts and circumstances of a major crime before the Lines of Enquiry are chosen.

Following that stage of an investigation, it is then the responsibility of the Senior Investigating Officer to select a Management Team. Each member should be chosen on the basis of individual skills required to manage each investigative area identified within the Lines of Enquiry. It is then the responsibility of the members of the Management Team to ensure that their designated areas of enquiry are thoroughly investigated.

In recent years it has become popular for senior detectives to organise 'Brainstorming Sessions' with other senior officers. From such meetings, issues can be raised and innovative ideas put forward. The list below is a sample of what could be considered now as Lines of Enquiry following the discovery of the fourth Ripper victim.

1. The Scene

Both scenes would be cordoned off and handed to forensic teams to examine in minute detail. Items such as blood or other human fluids or tissue would be sought, together with clothing fibres or other articles which may have been left by the killer.

2. The Murder Weapon

Any description of the murder weapon would be considered with previous descriptions. Assistance would be obtained from the Home Office pathologist who performed the post mortems on Stride and Eddowes. The most accurate detail of the instrument responsible for the murders would then be circulated to the operational police officers and search teams formed to examine the most likely escape route used by the murderer. Certainly the areas linking Berner Street with Mitre Square would be subjected to detailed examination, as would those linking Mitre Square with Goulston Street and Dorset Street.

3. House to House Enquiries

Teams of officers would be tasked with making enquiries in the localities of both murder scenes, with a view to tracing witnesses and obtaining any intelligence likely to assist the investigation. Again, as with the search teams, those streets linking the locations known to have been visited by the killer would be subjected to enquiries by these officers.

4. Tasked Informants

Individual informants used by the police to obtain intelligence would be tasked with providing positive information which could help identify the killer.

5. Press and Media

Appeals for assistance from the public would be made through the media. Any descriptions of the murder weapon or suspects would be released for general knowledge.

6. Crime Pattern Analysis

Intelligence analysts would be requested to develop Sequence of Events Charts, liaising with the analyst already engaged on the previous two murders. The charts would show the last known movements of the victims prior to their deaths. Victim Profiles would be completed and any unusual factors identified.

7. Hospital Enquiries

As with the previous Ripper murders, general hospitals would be visited, to try and confirm whether any person had sought medical assistance immediately after the murders had been committed. The killer could have sustained injuries from the victims or been responsible for injuring himself accidentally during the attacks. Because of the nature of the crimes, records would be examined at mental hospitals to identify individuals who could have escaped from secure accommodation or been on temporary leave, particularly those who would be residing in areas close to Whitechapel.

It is important for a senior investigating officer to restrict an investigation to a size which can be effectively managed. The Lines of Enquiry should remain limited and not be affected by red herrings, which can create a wider base for the investigation to sit upon. The more confined the enquiry parameters are, the stronger the investigation will be and the likelihood of success increased.

Five

Police Versus the Press

Relationships between senior investigating officers and the news media can on occasions be akin to a turbulent romance. Both parties need a level of mutual understanding of each other's requirements. For officers in charge of a major enquiry, the press can be an important vehicle upon which appeals for help from the general public can be carried. At the same time, the media require information and material upon which to base their news items. Unfortunately there are occasions when demands from both sides are not met, and frustration and animosity result.

When a senior investigating officer refuses to disclose any detail whatsoever, then constant pestering and occasional bullying by individual journalists desperate for information can occur. Alternatively, reporters who attempt to reinforce their own critical opinions and judgements on police performances, by inaccurately reporting facts given to them, can also be subjected to a degree of retribution. There have been many occasions when individuals have found themselves isolated from the flow of information being provided by the police. In all high-profile cases such as the Ripper murders, there is a need for skilful handling of the media, which normally comes from understanding the requirements of those who are responsible for communicating news to the public.

Although the principal requirement for a senior investigating officer is to concentrate energy and attention towards the management of an investigation, it is also important that the requirements of the media are recognized. The majority of newspapers, television and radio stations accept that it is difficult for the officer in charge of a murder investigation to allocate a great deal of time to their reporters. However, they justifiably ask to be treated respectfully in return for the assistance they the media can give to a major enquiry.

In the majority of cases it is good practice for the senior police officer to chair a formal press conference and allow questions to be asked. The answers should be open and truthful, and as much information as possible should be shared with the public. Where there are sensitive areas in which, for whatever reason, public disclosure could be detrimental to an enquiry, then it is the responsibility of the police to protect that confidentiality. However, in those circumstances it should also be made clear to journalists the reasons for not divulging certain information. There are favourite phrases frequently used to deflect specific enquiries that do cause irritation and can project, quite wrongly, sinister evasiveness.

Disappointment and on occasions even friction can be created by the words 'No comment' or 'I'm not prepared to discuss that', given in answer to a question or valid point made by a reporter asking a question or making a point that is in the public interest. Where a situation exists which dictates limited disclosure, it is far better to reply truthfully 'I am sorry, but at the moment I cannot disclose that information because it's not in the best interests of my enquiries to do so', or 'We are making enquiries along those lines, but at the moment I cannot assist you any further because of the sensitivity of what my officers are doing'.

The majority of police forces today have a Press Office from which statements can be released. Trained and experienced press liaison officers are allocated to senior investigating officers to support and assist in dealing with the media. However, reporters still prefer interviews with the person leading the investigation, and on occasions it is essential to maintain public interest in a specific case. It is usual for a senior investigating officer to allow personal interviews to take place periodically, leaving the daily responsibilities for press liaison to those who are employed for that purpose.

There are occasions when an incident occurs or a situation arises during an investigation which the senior detective needs to share with the public. It may be that the enquiry requires some form of stimulus to rekindle public interest, or to help to trace a person or object. In either of those circumstances a statement should be channelled through the Force Press Office or a further press conference called. It is not good practice to completely ignore members of the media, expecting them to go away.

In instances where reporters have been starved of information, newspapers have been known to create their own stories which have partly been fictitious. Whether such practices have resulted from naïvety or been created by design is not important. The difficulties that can result from false information being fed to the public can be detrimental to an investigation and occasionally embarrassing. A typical example is when members of the press learn that a description of an offender has come into the possession of the police and are informed that an artist's impression will be released as soon as possible. There have been incidents when impatience has overtaken empathy and newspapers have arranged to have their own artist's impression created and printed before the official version has been formally released to them. The dangers of such a practice are obvious. In the majority of cases the newspaper print will bear no resemblance whatsoever to the one obtained from the evidence of eyewitnesses. Understandably, the public will consider and digest the details of the first picture published, only to become confused when the official and more accurate picture is released.

Relationships between police and press depend very much on the individuals involved. A number of senior investigating officers have enjoyed excellent relationships with journalists and have had little difficulty in cultivating effective and professional lines of communication. Problems can sometimes exist when those lines of communication stretch to four different sections of the media. The local newspapers work and perform differently from those journalists employed by national newspapers. Television and radio are separate facilities provided by different organizations or different departments within the same organization. The experienced senior investigating officer will have developed sound relationships with representatives from all of the four media areas, but the less experienced officer may only have knowledge of a few local reporters, or perhaps none at all.

Detective Superintendent Abberline informed his Management Team that he had agreed to hold a press conference at Scotland Yard at 11.00 a.m. on Monday, 1 October 1888, the day after the murders of Elizabeth Stride and Catharine Eddowes. Others who were to be present included Detective Chief Superintendent Arnold and Miss Betty McGuire, the force press liaison officer. A number of his senior managers had previously agreed with him that appeals for public help were required and needed to be made. Also it was important to try and reassure the public, particularly those living in Whitechapel, that the police were doing everything they possibly could to capture the murderer.

There were mixed feelings at the Management Team meeting as to whether or not Abberline should release the descriptions given by witnesses who saw Stride talking to a man just prior to her murder. Some members of the team thought that the information should not be made public until they were certain there were no more details to be obtained. They were hoping for other witnesses to come forward with better descriptions, following the general public appeals for help made through the media. Others had showed some doubt as to whether Elizabeth Stride's killer was the same person responsible for the murders of Nichols, Chapman and Eddowes, and didn't think it wise to publicly link the crimes at such an early stage. Abberline discussed his own views with his team and thought carefully about the course of action he should take. He decided that the absence of any description could provoke newspapers and television companies into creating their own. He decided to release the composite description which had been forwarded for circulation in the *Police Gazette*.

There had been a lot of comings and goings on the third floor where the press conference was to take place. Television crews with their lighting, camera and sound equipment had been clattering up and down stairs, accompanied by the sound of numerous press reporters holding conversations on mobile phones, seemingly all at the same time. Abberline walked into the long narrow room and sat between Arnold and McGuire, who had already taken up their positions behind a table upon which microphones had been carefully placed. He looked directly into the glaring lights which were pointing towards him, there for the benefit of three television cameras present. Behind those were approximately 50 reporters all seated on rows of chairs, each holding notepads and writing implements. A young woman was crouched on the floor just in front of the desk at which Abberline sat, holding a microphone up towards him, ready to capture every spoken word on tape.

After allowing time for his eyes to become adjusted to the lights, Abberline wished everyone a good morning and asked whether they had taken the opportunity to participate in the coffee and biscuits provided. The refreshments were there to present a warm and friendly welcome to those in attendance, but looking at the hungry sea of faces staring back at him, he realized that news was the only real commodity that would satisfy them.

The senior officer introduced his two colleagues and, looking down at a piece of paper in front of him, read the following statement:

'During the early hours of last Sunday morning the body of a female in her mid-forties was found in Berner Street, Whitechapel. She had been brutally murdered, and we are appealing for any person who was in that area between 11.30 on the evening of Saturday, 29 September, and 1.00 the following morning, and saw anyone or anything that was suspicious, to come forward.

At 1.45 the same morning, another female, who was again in her mid-forties, was found murdered in Mitre Square, Whitechapel. We are appealing for any person who was in the Square between 1.00 and when the murder was discovered, and saw anyone or anything suspicious, to come forward.

Both women had their throats cut by a sharp instrument, probably a knife with a long, narrow blade. The two bodies have been formally identified. The first murder victim found in Berner Street is known by the name of Elizabeth Stride, who we believe is of no fixed address. The murdered woman found in Mitre Square is a woman known by the name of Catharine Eddowes who, like the first victim, had no fixed address as far as we are aware.

We want to trace a man who was seen in Berner Street between 12.35 a.m. and 12.45 a.m. He is aged between twenty-eight and thirty years. He is between five foot five inches and five foot eight inches tall, with a fair to dark complexion. The man had dark hair and a small dark moustache, with a full face, and was broad-shouldered. He was thought to have been

wearing a dark diagonal coat and dark trousers. We also believe
that he had a collar and tie and was wearing a felt hat, possibly
black in colour. He was seen carrying something wrapped up in
newspaper. Are there any questions?'

Abberline had deliberately held back any information
concerning the victims' addresses or names of relatives, to try
and limit the amount of aggravation reporters can sometimes
cause innocent people.

'Superintendent, will you be leading both murder enquiries?'

'Yes.'

'Are they the work of Jack the Ripper?'

'It's too early to say at the moment, but there is a strong
possibility and we are making the necessary enquiries to
ascertain whether or not they are linked to the Ripper enquiries.'

'Whereabouts in Berner Street was the body found? We
understand that she was inside the gateway to a Working Men's
Club there?'

'Yes she was.'

'Who found the first body?'

Abberline knew that the reporters had already visited the
scene of the first murder and would be aware of the witness
Diemschutz and his involvement.

'A Mr Diemschutz, the steward of the club.'

'Were there any other injuries to the first woman apart from
the cut throat?'

'No.'

'Who found the second body?'

'A patrolling police officer.'

'Can we interview that officer?'

'No.'

'Can you give us his name?'

'No, I don't want to expose him at the moment. He is a
young uniformed officer who was walking his beat, which

101

included Mitre Square on that particular night. I am extremely pleased with the way in which he dealt with what really was a terrifying incident for him.'

'Where are the bodies now?'

'In the Central Mortuary under police guard.'

One female reporter seated at the very back of the room shouted out the next question.

'Are you linking these two murders?'

Arnold interrupted before Abberline could answer. 'Yes, for the time being.'

'Why?'

Arnold remained silent and Abberline answered. 'Because both women had been killed in the same way and the murders were committed only a few hundred yards from each other. If we find evidence to show that different people were involved, then we shall treat them separately, but at the moment I think it's safe to assume that the same person was responsible for both murders.'

'Were there any other injuries on the second woman?'

Abberline paused and then said, 'Yes, other parts of her body had been violated.'

'What do you mean by that? Had she been sexually attacked?'

'It's too early to say at the moment whether there was a sexual motive in either of the cases.'

'Had the second woman been mutilated?'

'Yes.'

There was a short period of time when everyone in the room seemed to look and whisper between each other. Certainly for a moment, an air of excitement filled the room.

'Superintendent, were the mutilations on the second woman similar to those on the first two murders?'

'I'm not in a position to disclose that information at the moment, but if you're asking me whether I believe that the two murders that occurred yesterday were committed by the same man responsible for the murders of Polly Nichols and Annie Chapman, then I would have to say that we are looking into that possibility.'

'Is it possible then that the Ripper was disturbed by Mr Diemschutz and that's why she only had her throat cut?'

'At the moment I am not saying that these two murders were the work of the Ripper, but yes, what you suggest is possible.'

'If you're not sure that the Ripper was responsible for the murders on Sunday, why are you dealing with them instead of the local police?'

Arnold again interrupted. 'Detective Superintendent Abberline is the officer in charge of the Chapman and Nichols investigations. Because of the possible links to those murders, he will conduct the enquiries into Stride and Eddowes.'

'How many officers have you got working on all of the investigations at the moment?'

Abberline replied, 'About a hundred.'

'Have you any leads yet?'

'We have a number of leads from each of the murders, and I have officers working on them whilst we speak.' Abberline knew that sooner or later he would have to give the press something more positive, if he was to avoid further criticism and help ease the unrest that was now growing stronger amongst the Whitechapel residents.

'Is there anything you wish to say to the people of Whitechapel about the murders?'

Again Abberline paused and thought before he spoke. 'Yes, there is. Let me assure everyone that we are doing everything possible to catch the person responsible for these murders. Myself and my investigation team are optimistic that we shall bring him to justice.'

'What about the women in Whitechapel who are frightened to death to walk on the streets at night?'

'They have every right to be, but it's no good people becoming alarmed. I would suggest that until we have caught the killer women should stay off the streets during the hours of darkness, or make sure they are accompanied by a male who is known to them.'

'Is it not right, Mr Abberline, that the police are losing control of Whitechapel because of your failure to catch the Ripper?'

'I do not agree with that suggestion. The police are in control and will remain so. All I ask the public to be is patient until we've got him behind bars. There are a number of on-going operations to reduce the risk to women, but I am not prepared to disclose the details of them for obvious reasons.'

'Don't you think you should tell the public what you are doing? Don't you think that they deserve to know what their police are doing to protect them?'

'I am not prepared to let the killer know what we are doing to try and catch him. I don't want him to be frightened away.' Abberline immediately knew that he had made a mistake and wanted to retract that last statement, but it was too late.

Three reporters spoke at the same time and were asked by the press liaison officer to restrict their questions to one at a time.

'Mr Abberline, you believe then that the Ripper should be encouraged to return to Whitechapel and try and kill again?'

Abberline now wished a hole in the floor would open up so that he could dive into it.

'I'm not saying that. We are doing all we can to catch him, and we are optimistic that we shall have him sooner rather than later. People need not be alarmed but need to be cautious, particularly at night.'

'Were the last two victims prostitutes?'

That question gave Abberline some respite and he paused for quite some time before answering. 'Yes, I believe so.'

'Mr Abberline, do you know how much these investigations have cost so far?'

'Yes, but there are no financial limitations at present. We are pulling out all the stops to catch this killer, and the financial implications will be secondary until we have caught him.'

'Are you arranging for an artist's impression of the killer?'

'I am optimistic that we might have something to release to you in the next few days.'

'How many witnesses have you interviewed so far that have seen him?'

Abberline paused again before answering. 'There are a number of people who have been interviewed and provided us with valuable information. There are still witnesses to be seen, and I am hoping that when we have collated all the information together, we might have a picture worth circulating.'

'Will you be doing a computer composite of the killer?'

'That is a possibility, but we shall have to see. I can assure you that if and when we obtain sufficient material to complete one, you will be the first to know.'

'Is it right that you suspect that the killer is a doctor?'

'I am not in the practice of making suppositions. I only deal with facts, and until we are in a position to have the full picture, which I am sure will evolve from our enquiries, then I must avoid conjecture.'

'But surely it is more than conjecture. The way in which these women were attacked leads people to believe that the killer must have had some medical knowledge. Is that not correct?'

Abberline glared towards the reporter who had asked the question and snapped, 'Conjecture, my friend, only conjecture at the moment.' He then nodded towards McGuire, which was the signal to bring the press conference to an end. A number of television and radio reporters requested 'one to one' interviews with the Senior Investigating Officer, and he agreed.

Thirty minutes later, Abberline was sitting at his own desk facing Arnold, who was standing over him. Both men were fairly satisfied at the way in which they had handled the press conference, although they agreed with each other that what they had just experienced was similar to sitting in an overheated Turkish Bath. Arnold made a comment about the error Abberline had made in misleading reporters into believing that he wanted the Ripper to continue visiting Whitechapel. Abberline just shook his head and nothing more was said about that specific point. Arnold also queried why Abberline had declined to allow PC Watkins to be interviewed about finding Eddowes' body. He thought that putting the young officer up as a hero would have given the reporters something more positive from the police point of view. Abberline didn't agree and explained that his main concern was that the young officer could have innocently disclosed information that they didn't want the public or murderer to know about.

Both men returned to their individual duties, Abberline calling for a carriage to return to the scenes in Berner Street and Mitre Square, and Arnold making his way towards the Commissioner's office to update him. Until she received further instructions, Betty McGuire would now take on the responsibility of dealing with press enquiries on a day to day basis.

Six

The Twenty-eight-day Review

Abberline's office resembled a Victorian drawing-room rather than a clerical work station. A large black grate surrounded by a deep red tiled hearth constantly fostered a bright glowing coal fire throughout the winter months, throwing shadows across highly polished floorboards and occasionally spitting hot embers at the woollen rugs. There were many occasions when the policeman's only companion was the warmth and friendly face of the burning coals. Many of his deepest thoughts would become dislodged and easily extracted from the profound craters of his mind whilst he stared into the flames, momentarily isolated from the rest of the world and unaware of the remainder of his surroundings. The crimson relief of the heavy flocked wallpaper seemed to be more defined by the light shining from the two gas lamps fitted either side of the hearth. The three woollen floor rugs complemented the red leather upholstery of two roundbacked chairs facing his solid oak desk. The atmosphere was warm, pleasant and homely; ideal for the long hours he usually spent working there.

During the days that immediately followed the double murders of Stride and Eddowes, Abberline's office comforts were tested to the limit. His private and confidential room, his chosen retreat, with pictures of past friends and colleagues adorning its walls, was slowly becoming something similar to a circus arena and he strongly objected, but to no avail. At one stage there appeared to be a constant flow of police officers and support staff members, who had been requested to assist the Review Team, walking in and out of his office, constantly questioning and badgering him, demanding immediate answers. The reviewing officer, Detective Chief Superintendent Arnold, eventually decided to share the office, much to Abberline's displeasure. On occasions the junior officer wondered whether his senior had left home to live there.

As the hours, days and nights passed by, friction between the two senior detectives began to dominate their professional relationship. Both men were autocratic by nature and found it easier to talk at one another rather than listen to each other's views, if they didn't comply with their own. Their receptive skills required much improvement, and for long periods of time they resembled two opposing magnetic poles, pushing against each other.

On the third day of the Review Arnold and Abberline found themselves in the Commissioner's office. Sir Charles Warren had been subjected to increasing pressure from a number of Whitehall officials and members of the government, including the Prime Minister and Home Secretary. He begged both senior detectives to 'work as one' and focus all of their investigative experience and knowledge on the task that lay in front of them.

'I must have him now, gentlemen. The East End is becoming very difficult and other people, far more powerful than I, are demanding this monster's capture.'

Abberline sarcastically asked whether the Commissioner wanted the Ripper caught, or would anyone do? Arnold glared at his junior officer and Sir Charles replied, 'Gentlemen, either we catch him or we fail. If we fail, then I do not think any of us will be here in a month's time. Never has the challenge been so great, but this government cannot afford any further disorder in London. It stands on the brink of going to the country again, and the Ripper murders are helping to push it there.' The two CID officers accepted their admonishment and left grim-faced.

Abberline stood behind his desk looking across the autumn sky towards St Paul's Cathedral. He thought of how foolish he must have looked and deeply regretted his cynicism towards the Commissioner. Arnold entered the room and made his presence felt by slamming a bundle of papers on top of the desk he had arranged to have moved into Abberline's office at the commencement of the Review. Abberline remained stationary, still gazing out of the window. It was a good time to iron out their difficulties.

'He wants the Review completed by the end of the week now, Fred.'

'Then he must have it,' replied Abberline.

'We need to talk, Fred; we need to work more amicably together to crack this one. We both want the same result, and dammit, we are the best in the country and should be capable of catching this bastard.'

Abberline agreed with his senior officer, wondering whether the pressures of constant demands and stresses over the past few weeks had somewhat clouded his own judgement and thinking ability. Both senior officers agreed to forget their differences and concentrate wholly on working together as a team, both with the one same objective: to catch the Ripper.

After the meeting with the Commissioner, the next 48 hours were fruitful. Both senior detectives examined, analysed and discussed every detail and aspect of the investigations. They partnered each other in a more convivial atmosphere, although more from necessity rather than personal choice, but the job was done and completed in the most efficient and effective way.

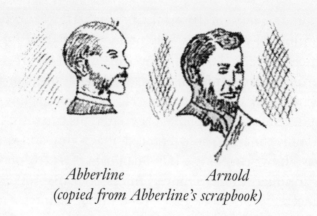

Abberline   *Arnold*
(copied from Abberline's scrapbook)

The common objective of reviewing any undetected major crime is to assist and support the Senior Investigating Officer in trying to identify the offender and eventually secure a conviction. In addition, it is important that good and bad practices are identified by the Review Team for the purposes of assisting similar investigations in the future.

There are a number of guidelines for police forces to follow, although it is a matter for individual forces as to how a Review Team is structured. In normal circumstances the rank of the Reviewing Officer should be at least the same as that of the Senior Investigating Officer who is in charge of the major crime enquiry. This is to avoid any embarrassment between the two officers. It would be improper and impractical for a junior ranking officer to be given the responsibility of inspecting the work of a senior.

The Review Team should also include a computer operator, preferably a supervisor, who has the ability to examine data. Other members of the team should possess various skills and experience in the specific areas allocated to them for inspection.

At the commencement of a Review, the Senior Investigating Officer should fully brief the Review Team and perhaps arrange for them to visit the scene, or as in the case of the Ripper murders, all of the scenes, as soon as possible. The Reviewing

Officer should have been previously supplied with copies of the Policy File, logs of events and statements obtained from the main witnesses. This would enable members of the Review Team to be fully conversant with the investigation before commencement of the Review.

It is essential that during a Review, the Senior Investigating Officer and his Management Team are kept fully aware of any problems or suggestions made by members of the Review Team. Regular meetings can achieve this and assist in maintaining good liaison and relationships.

Arnold knew that there was an urgent need to reduce the level of public concern, and the Commissioner needed new material to throw to the wolves who were baying for his blood. He drove his Review Team to complete the inspection with energy and in haste. They virtually worked around the clock on the Chief Superintendent's instructions. In the majority of cases involving four homicides, a Review could take up to a month or longer to complete. Arnold was determined to deliver his final report within a week of the Review commencing. He was fully aware of what the objectives should be, but also had a personal desire to identify ways and methods of improving the likelihood of success. Operational matters were to take precedent over administrative issues.

The terms of reference given to each reviewing officer usually relate to the areas of the investigation to be examined. In most cases they will include the following:

A Press File should have been maintained throughout the investigation, and a member of the Review Team would be responsible for examining it to ensure the media had been used to maximum effect. All documentation relevant to the selected Lines of Enquiry should also be scrutinized and additional subjects identified, if the Reviewing Officer thought it necessary to expedite enquiries. These particular areas should be researched in depth by the Review Team. There are other parts of the investigation which would obviously need to be examined. However, a general picture of the levels of efficiency being practised in the Major Incident Room could be obtained by means of 'dip sampling' material and analysing it, rather than waste time inspecting every piece of work completed.

It is also important that members of the Review Team hold regular debriefs with police officers and support staff engaged on the enquiry. Both the Senior Investigating Officer and the Office Manager responsible for the running of the MIR should be consulted on a regular basis.

Each member of the Review Team should then submit a report outlining their results and recommendations to the Reviewing Officer, who will compile a composite document for the information of the Commissioner or Chief of Police.

On 6 October the following report was handed to Sir Charles Warren:

METROPOLITAN POLICE

6 October 1888

TO: The Commissioner of Police
FROM: Detective Chief Superintendent Arnold
         Head of Criminal Investigation Department

SUBJECT: Review of the Whitechapel Murders

Sir,
Between 30 September and 5 October 1888 a Review of the following investigations currently being conducted in the Whitechapel area was completed by myself.

1. Mary Ann Nichols – murdered in Bucks Row on 31 August 1888.

2. Annie May Chapman – murdered in Hanbury Street on 8 September 1888.

3. Elizabeth Stride – murdered in Berner Street on 30 September 1888.

4. Catharine Eddowes – murdered in Mitre Square on 30 September 1888.

The Review Team are listed below together with the nominated areas allocated to each member for their inspection.

Detective Chief Superintendent Arnold –	Policy and Strategy.
Detective Inspector Burton –	Computer Database and System.
Miss Aldritt –	Finance Officer.
Detective Sergeant Wallis –	Welfare and Resource Issues.

The Review Team examined the following areas and the results are as reported.

General Background

The current situation is that the first two murders are being investigated as separate enquiries, each having a senior investigating officer in charge. Detective Superintendent Abberline is the senior officer in overall command. The second two murders have been linked together and are being investigated as a separate enquiry to the previous two murders but under the command of Mr Abberline.

There are currently three Major Incident Rooms, one for each of the Nichols and Chapman murders and the third for the linked enquiry into the deaths of Stride and Eddowes. All three MIRs are supported by a computer database and financed from Central Contingency Funds maintained at Scotland Yard.

There are Intelligence Cells attached to each MIR and co-ordinated by a central computer facility which is networked to each investigation. This allows the senior investigating officers computer access to all of the investigations.

Policy and Structure

The Commanding Officer, Detective Superintendent Abberline, has maintained Policy Files for each investigation. They were found to be current and had been completed on a daily basis. Each file recorded all policy decisions made including the type of scene examinations; results of post mortems; Lines of Enquiry; selected members of the Management Team and strategy plans. Budgetary and financial considerations were also properly recorded, together with the number of personnel deployed on the overall enquiries.

The current total number of resources being used are outlined in Appendix One together with the centralized support resources.

The total number of police and support staff is currently 125.

Lines of Enquiry

The following Lines of Enquiry are currently being investigated in all of the murder enquiries:

1. Investigation of the scene.

2. House to house enquiries.

3. Profiles of the victim and suspect.

114

4. Hospital enquiries.

5. Cabs and hansom fares.

6. Merchant Navy ships and crews visiting the London Docks.

7. Press and media.

The Investigation Teams responsible for the Nichols and Chapman enquiries are also examining the following additional Lines of Enquiry:

1. Crime Pattern Analysis.

2. Boot prints found at both scenes.

3. Dyed woollen fibres found at both scenes.

4. Enquiries with the medical profession.

5. Intelligence received from professional informants.

Crisis Management and Think Tanks
Crisis Management Meetings have followed the discovery of each murder. All have been chaired by Detective Superintendent Abberline and sound strategical plans have resulted. Also, Mr Abberline has periodically organized a number of Think Tanks which have helped to strengthen the Management Teams and given added direction to the investigations. A number of non-police personnel have also been invited to attend, including lawyers, members from the medical profession and Local Authority departments.

Senior officers from across the force have participated in each exercise and helped to produce a number of objective and innovative ideas ensuring that all options have been considered. Members of the National Crime Faculty, who are responsible for recording and monitoring undetected murder investigations on a national basis, have also attended and inputted relevant information and suggestions.

Finance
The current situation is that payment for a total of 6,000 working police hours has been contributed towards the investigations from central funds. The budgetary records were found to be in order and it is suggested that further financial support should be provided in the near future. It is recommended that a further payment for 1,000 working police hours be allocated to the Commanding Officer forthwith and future financial reviews take place on a weekly basis.

Victim Support
In all four murders being investigated, there have been difficulties in tracing known relatives and associates of victims. Where there has been some success, trained police officers have been tasked with supporting and counselling on a long-term basis.

The Computer Database
The three Major Incident Rooms currently in operation were found to be fully updated with the information inputted into the computer system. Information had been correctly recorded into appropriate categories and the majority of the number of enquiries allocated to outside crews for investigation, had been completed (71%). The Review Team could not find any discrepancies.

Welfare Issues

Four weeks have now passed since the murder of Mary Ann Nichols, and there are a number of officers who have been engaged on that investigation since it commenced. Counselling and support facilities for people requesting assistance have been made available. Following the discovery of the Eddowes murder, three officers have reported sick with stress and psychological problems. Those officers are being monitored by the Senior Management Team.

Records showing officers' time off and leave from duty have also been examined and each officer is now required to take a minimum of 48 hours' leave during each weekly period. Designated hours of working do not exceed eight hours a day unless exceptional circumstances exist.

Recommendations

Having consulted with Detective Superintendent Abberline and his Management Teams, there has been general agreement for the need to reduce the investigation parameters. The number of resources will also be refined by linking all four murder investigations, which could then be managed from one central site. The recommended structure is outlined in Appendix Two.

One computer database would be required, which would be managed from a centralized site. The staffing levels for the investigation would be reduced from the current 125 to 115, which would include the following additional intelligence and press support staff.

> 1 x Det. Sergeant
> 6 x Det. Constables (Intelligence Operatives)
> 3 x Intelligence Analysts
> 1 x Press Officer

The Review Team also recommend that the following Lines of Enquiry now take precedence in directing future investi-

117

gations. Again, these have been selected following consultation with Detective Superintendent Abberline and his Management Teams.

1. Investigation of the scenes and enquiries resulting from forensic examinations.

2. Profiles of the victim and suspect.

3. Hospital enquiries to be continued.

4. All hackney carriage coachmen working in the Whitechapel area to be seen regarding fares transported into the relevant areas on the dates in question.

5. Merchant Navy ships and crews visiting the London Docks on the dates of the murders to be traced.

6. Effective use of the press and media.

7. Enquiries to continue relevant to the boot print found at both scenes.

8. Enquiries to continue relevant to the dyed woollen fibres found at both scenes.

9. Enquiries to continue with members of the medical profession.

10. Professional informants to be tasked with obtaining information relevant to the investigation.

(signed) G Arnold
Detective Chief Superintendent

Appendix One

Current Resources:

Nichols Enquiry

Operational Crews
1 x Det. Chief Inspector
1 x Det. Inspector
2 x Det. Sergeants
12 x Det. Constables

Intelligence Cell
1 x Det. Sergeant
2 x Det. Constables
1 x Analyst

Incident Room Staff
1 x Det. Sergeant (Statement Reader)
1 x Det. Constable (Exhibits Officer)
2 x Computer Inputters
1 x Typists
1 x Clerical Assistants

Chapman Enquiry

Operational Crews
1 x Det. Chief Inspector
1 x Det. Inspector
3 x Det. Sergeants
18 x Det. Constables

Intelligence Cell
1 x Det. Sergeant
2 x Det. Constables
1 x Analyst

Incident Room Staff
1 x Det. Sergeant (Statement Reader)
1 x Det. Constable (Exhibits Officer)
3 x Computer Inputters
2 x Typists
2 x Clerical Assistants

THE WHITECHAPEL MURDERS – SOLVED?

Stride and Eddowes Enquiries

Operational Crews
- 1 x Det. Chief Inspector
- 2 x Det. Inspector
- 4 x Det. Sergeants
- 24 x Det. Constables

Intelligence Cell
- 1 x Det. Sergeant
- 3 x Det. Constables
- 1 x Analyst

Incident Room Staff
- 2 x Det. Sergeant (Statement Reader)
- 1 x Det. Constable (Exhibits Officer)
- 4 x Computer Inputters
- 3 x Typists
- 2 x Clerical Assistants

Centralised Support Resources
- 1 x Detective Inspector (Co-ordinating Officer)
- 6 x Detective Constables (Intelligence Officers)
- 4 x Scenes of Crime Officers
- 2 x Plan Drawers
- 2 x Press Liaison Officers

Appendix Two

1. *Nichols Enquiry*	2. *Chapman Enquiry*
Investigation Crews	Investigation Crews
1 x Det. Inspector	1 x Det. Inspector
2 x Det. Sergeants	2 x Det. Sergeants
12 x Det. Constables	12 x Det. Constables

Central Support
Management Team
Det. Superintendent Abberline
1 x Det. Chief Inspector (Operations)
1 x Det. Chief Inspector (Support/Intelligence)
1 x Det. Inspector (Scenes of Crime)
1 x Forensic Scientist (Laboratory liaison)
1 x Administration Officer
1 x Financial Officer
1 x Welfare Officer

Major Incident Room
1 x Det. Chief Inspector
1 x Det. Inspector
4 x Det. Sergeants
4 x Det. Constables

(Exhibits and Scenes of Crime liaison)
10 x Inputters
10 x Typists
6 x Clerical Assistants

3. *Stride Enquiry*	4. *Eddowes Enquiry*
Investigation Crews	Investigation Crews
1 x Det. Inspector	1 x Det. Inspector
2 x Det. Sergeants	2 x Det. Sergeants
12 x Det. Constables	12 x Det. Constables

On the evening of 6 October, Arnold and Abberline were summoned to the Commissioner's office and the Review Report was discussed in detail. Perhaps for the first time in weeks, Sir Charles Warren looked a little more optimistic. He asked both men if they believed the Ripper would be caught sooner rather than later. Arnold was optimistic in his reply and made it clear that he believed the net was closing in on the murderer. Abberline was less enthusiastic and voiced his fears that the killer could strike again. He suggested that more increased beat patrols would assist in preventing further murders being committed.

The Commissioner agreed to implement the recommendations included in Arnold's report and instructed more beat patrol officers be transferred to the Whitechapel district to perform night duty. He also suggested that policewomen supported by teams of male officers be used as decoys in the red light district. He concluded the meeting with the following words, 'One more death, gentlemen, and I do believe we shall all be hung out to dry.'

Abberline had little sleep that night, and the following day he returned to visit Mitre Square, where for a while he stood alone in silence. He carefully observed the many small passageways and alleys which ran off the square. He then followed a route along Duke Street into Aldgate and turned left into Goulston Street. He stopped near to where the piece of bloodstained apron had been found and gazed upon the clusters of terraced houses that ran both sides of the street. He still had difficulty in accepting that no one had seen or heard the killer's movements. He then made his way towards Dorset Street and stood near the public wash-basin where more bloodstains had been discovered. He sketched a map of the area he had walked connecting Mitre Square with Goulston Street and Dorset Street. The direction taken by the murderer from the scene of his last victim was north, away from Tower

Bridge and London Docks. Abberline felt that he was close to the Ripper; he needed one piece of luck to turn the whole enquiry on its head. He looked skywards and prayed for more inspiration before returning to the Yard.

Abberline pinned the sketch-map to his office wall. He then sent for a local street map which included the whole area and pinned that next to his own. The officer knew most of Whitechapel intimately, having worked there as a detective for the previous 14 years, before transferring to where he now sat. He looked closely at both the map and sketch, as though waiting for answers to a number of questions to jump out in front of him. Abberline believed the man he was hunting was both intelligent and cunning. He suspected that the clues left by the Ripper, the bloodstained apron and writing on the wall, together with bloodstains around the wash-basin, had been left deliberately as decoys. They all indicated an escape route north of where Eddowes had been murdered. 'Too convenient,' thought the investigator. 'Too bloody convenient by far.'

Abberline looked in the opposite direction, to the south of Mitre Square, where any further progress in escaping would have been halted by the docks, unless the killer crossed Tower Bridge or had access to one of the ships docked there. He was satisfied that the boot prints left at both of the first two murders hadn't been left by the killer deliberately, so they represented a real clue. He had been told that the boots responsible for the impressions had ridges cut by hand into the soles, a common practice with seamen. He drew a circle around the area of the docks.

The senior detective immediately telephoned downstairs to the detective inspector in charge of the Intelligence Cell and instructed him to concentrate on shipping lines and traffic using London Docks at the time of each of the murders. Lists of ships moored on the appropriate dates together with details of crew members needed to be given top priority.

123

Could Abberline have suddenly put his finger on the right button? Could this be the piece of luck he knew that he would need if the killer was to be caught? London Docks suddenly took on a whole new meaning for him which he hadn't recognized before. Could that grim and featureless world be Jack the Ripper's hiding place? Could it be the place where he sat and planned his next murder? Where he kept his murderous tools hidden and waiting to be brought out onto the streets of Whitechapel whenever the urge drove him? Abberline knew that there hadn't been sufficient investigative work done on the docks up to now. He suddenly felt a surge of excitement pass through his body. Perhaps this was the breakthrough he needed? 'The bastard's been coming into Whitechapel from the docks.'

Arnold had returned earlier to his own office, which was situated in another part of the building. Abberline telephoned him and told his senior officer of his suspicions and the way in which his new assessment of the circumstances had developed. Arnold was guarded and responded with a degree of caution.

'Let's just keep it away from the Commissioner's ears for now, Fred.'

Seven

Mary Jane Kelly

'The victim's clothing was piled neatly upon a chair in the room'

Following the double murders on 30 September 1888, the climate throughout the East End of London reached fever pitch, and it was to be almost six weeks before another, the final and most violent atrocity, took place. Although the police activity was intensive, there had been little success and all attempts to catch the Ripper had been frustrated. People living in Whitechapel feared for their safety and had little confidence in what the police were trying to achieve.

The official investigations were hindered by the local newspapers printing articles about the 'Ripper letters'. Following the murders of Stride and Eddowes, the public were told of a letter that had been received by the Central News Agency in London just prior to 30 September. It was dated 25 September and postmarked 27 September 1888. The letter read as follows:

Dear Boss,
I keep on hearing the police have caught me but they won't fix me just yet. I have laughed when they look so clever and talk about being on the right track. That joke about Leather Apron gave me real fits. I am down on whores and I shan't quit ripping them till I do get buckled. Grand work the last job was [Chapman]. *I gave*

125

the lady no time to squeal. How can they catch me now. I love my work and want to start again. You will soon hear of me with my funny little games. I saved some of the proper red stuff in a ginger beer bottle over the last job to write with but it went thick like glue and I can't use it. Red ink is fit enough I hope ha ha. *The next job I do I shall clip the lady's ears off and send to the police officers just for jolly wouldn't you. Keep this letter back till I do a bit more work, then give it out straight. My knife is nice and sharp I want to get to work right away if I get a chance. Good luck.*

Yours truly

JACK THE RIPPER

Don't mind me giving the trade name.

    Wasn't good enough to post this before I got all the red ink off my hands curse it. No luck yet they say I am a doctor now ha ha.

What is significant is that Eddowes' ears had been badly mutilated, although they had not been removed completely from her head.

On 1 October 1888, the day following the Stride and Eddowes murders, the same News Agency received another letter.

I was not codding dear old Boss when I gave you the tip. You'll hear about Saucy Jack's work tomorrow. Double event this time. Number one squealed a bit. Couldn't finish straight off. Had not time to get ears for police. Thanks for keeping last letter back till I got to work again.

JACK THE RIPPER

Details of the double murders were made public on 1 October 1888, which meant that anyone could have written the second note. However, reference to the 'ears' and the obvious attempt to remove those belonging to Catharine Eddowes, gave the letters some credibility.

George Lusk was a 49-year-old activist who lived in Tollit Street, Whitechapel. After being elected president of the Whitechapel Vigilance Committee, he sought publicity by writing about the Ripper murders to *The Times* newspaper. On 16 October he received a letter accompanied by a 3-inch-square cardboard box wrapped in brown paper. The box contained half of a human kidney preserved in spirits of wine. The letter read as follows:

Mr Lusk   *From Hell*
Sir,
I send you half the Kidne I took from one woman prasarved it for you tother piece I fried and ate it was very nise. I may send you the bloody knif that took it out if you only wate a whil longer
                signed Catch me when you can
                                Mishter Lusk

The degree of violence used against Mary Jane Kelly went far beyond reasonable human understanding of how one person could treat another. It was the last recognized murder committed by Jack the Ripper, and the victim was subjected to more force than any of the previous four women.

Abberline and his team of investigators were aware that the attacks had intensified as the number of victims increased. There is one popular theory suggested by some observers and researchers who have studied in detail the Whitechapel murders: the person responsible for the outrages was trying to trace a prostitute by the name of Kelly, and his previous victims were killed as a result of mistaken identity. The accuracy of such an interpretation could have been supported by the extreme violence used against the last victim. However, that being the case, then the pattern of force used against each of the women victims doesn't appear to suggest that the murderer was looking for a particular person. It could be assumed that the same level of violence would have been used in each case, rather than increasing with each victim.

There have been few people since the Ripper murders subjected to such horrendous injuries as Mary Kelly. If the work of the Ripper prior to the discovery of Kelly's body had spread fear and anxiety through the country, the events that followed the final murder accelerated public concern towards breaking-point. The whole structure of law and order saw ridges created in its foundations, and the government of the day almost fell. The police and other officials involved in the investigations were regarded as failures and what little public support there was dwindled dramatically.

Kelly was a different kind of prostitute from the other victims in that she appeared to be educated, pretty and well-spoken. She was born in Ireland of Irish-Catholic parents and moved with her family to Wales, where her father worked as a foreman at an ironworks. At the age of 16 Mary was married to a local worker, who was killed in a works explosion soon after the marriage.

It didn't take long for Mary Jane to become known on the streets of Cardiff as a common prostitute. Her addiction to the drink that usually accompanied her trade soon became obvious: gin. It is believed she spent some time in France, possibly a few weeks, and was frequently heard to talk about visits to Paris. Although there appear to have been many rumours concerning children by Mary Kelly, none have been confirmed, and whether or not she had any whilst in France or London has never been verified.

Kelly first came to light in Whitechapel during the early part of 1888, when she lived with an unemployed labourer by the name of Joseph Barnett. It was accepted at the time that her prostitution was kept from Barnett, although the two regularly quarrelled about her drinking habits. At the end of October 1888 Barnett left Mary Kelly living in lodgings at 13 Dorset Street. The accommodation was less than basic and could only be approached by way of a courtyard, Miller's Court. It was a dark and dismal part of the neighbourhood, with six other squalid dwellings clustered around a small square. The area was mostly made up of lodging-houses where many of the homeless found shelter for a few coppers a night.

John McCarthy rented number 27 Dorset Street from which he sold candles, soap and oil. He also rented other premises which he sublet to mostly destitute people who spent most of their time raising sufficient funds to pay for their lodgings. Mary Kelly's flat was such an accommodation, rented to her by McCarthy for four shillings and sixpence a week. Unfortunately both Kelly and Barnett had fallen behind with their weekly rent, and on 9 November 1888 McCarthy sent his shop assistant Tom Bowyer to collect the outstanding rent.

A narrow archway led from Dorset Street into Miller's Court, where Kelly's lodging-house was on the right. It was one of the coldest days of the year. An icy wind had greeted the morning's first light, and Bowyer wrapped his arms around his shoulders to keep warm as he stood outside Kelly's address. He knocked on the door with a loud bang. His brass pocket-watch told him that the time was 10.45 a.m., and the rent collector felt that his journey away from the blazing coal fire he had left was a wasted one. There wasn't much chance of Kelly opening the door to pay rent money. He knocked again, but there was still no answer. Following a final attempt to get some response, Bowyer decided he was wasting his time and turned to leave. However, the coldness of the morning made him a little more alert than usual, and he noticed a broken window with a piece of dirty material hanging on the inside, giving the appearance of some kind of curtain. The rent collector pulled the material to one side and looked through the small window.

What Tom Bowyer saw through the clouded grimy window was to stay in his mind for the rest of his life. He felt his stomach turn over and cold sweat poured down his brow as he looked upon a human mess that 'represented' the body of Mary Jane Kelly lying in a large pool of blood on the bed. She was practically naked and lay on her back, with her face, terribly mutilated, turned towards him. The ears and nose had been severed, and her throat deeply cut from one side to the other nearly severing the head from the body. Her legs were splayed apart, and on the right thigh lay the victim's liver. The stomach and abdomen had been ripped open, the breasts sliced off, the lower portion of the body, including the uterus, cut cleanly out. There were burnt remnants of female clothing in the grate, and the victim's clothing was piled neatly upon a chair in the room.

Within an hour of the discovery Abberline, Arnold and Doctor Phillips, the divisional surgeon, were at the scene. Forced entry gave them access to the 12-foot-square room which contained a bed and bedside table, and a thorough examination of the scene commenced. What the two senior police officers witnessed forced them to leave the room for a short while, to be physically sick. Whilst outside recovering in the open air, Abberline looked upwards at the grey cloudy sky and uncontrollably shouted at the top of his voice condemnations of the man responsible for such carnage, 'The bastard! The dirty bastard!' He then turned his attention to a small crowd of neighbours who had gathered together in Miller's Court and screamed at two younger police officers to clear the area. 'Get this lot of nosy bastards out of here. What's in there is not for human eyes.' He turned to Arnold and asked, 'What's the Commissioner going to say about this, then?' He was placated by his senior officer. What neither of them knew was that Sir Charles Warren had tendered his resignation as Commissioner of the Metropolitan Police the previous day.

One of the younger police officers who first attended the scene of Mary Kelly's death was a detective named Dew who later, as a detective chief inspector, was involved in the arrest of Crippen. The young DC Dew found on a table by the bed small piles of flesh, neatly laid out: the victim's breasts, heart and kidneys.

The *Illustrated Police News* reported the incident as follows:

The throat had been cut right across with a knife, nearly severing the head from the body. The abdomen had been partially ripped open, and both of the breasts had been cut from the body, the left arm, like the head, hung to the body by the skin only. The nose had been cut off, the forehead skinned, and the thighs, down to the feet, stripped of the flesh. The abdomen had been slashed with a knife across downwards, and the liver and entrails wrenched away. The entrails and other portions of the frame were missing, but the liver, etc., it is said, were found placed between the feet of the poor victim. The flesh from the thighs and legs, together with the breasts and nose, had been placed by the murderer on the table, and one of the hands of the dead woman had been pushed in her stomach.

Kelly – An Hypothesis, One Hundred Years On

Abberline wept as he looked down at the shredded body lying on the mortuary slab. The pathologist assured him that the victim knew very little about what had happened to her, but from an investigative point of view, nothing positive came from the post mortem. The Senior Investigating Officer still searched for a motive, knowing that none of the previous Ripper murders had revealed one. He wondered what kind of maniac would commit such horrendous atrocities without a reason; or perhaps there was a reason which had yet to be identified.

Abberline instructed every person involved on the enquiry to attend the briefing that followed the post mortem. Because of this, an open space not far from Scotland Yard was used to accommodate the number of people who would be present. Security was a problem, particularly from the press and media, but the Senior Investigating Officer was not too concerned. From his point of view, anger was still clouding his judgement, and he knew that he had to quickly revert back to being the professional police officer he was, if the investigation was to continue with any useful purpose.

Abberline could see the levels of exhaustion showing on the pale, worn-out looks on the faces of the majority of officers and civilians who were in attendance for the briefing. The long and demanding enquiries had taken their toll, and Abberline appreciated the difficulties his people had been experiencing. He told them of his gratitude for what they had done and the pride he felt from their unrewarded and unselfish efforts. He tried to inject some stimulation and motivation into all concerned with a promise that the Ripper would be caught very soon, and he succeeded. He described the man they were searching for as, 'An evil person living amongst us that must be sought out and brought to justice'. He told the briefing that he wanted them to persist with those Lines of Enquiry already identified. An additional team of local CID and uniform officers would make the necessary enquiries into Kelly's murder and would work directly to himself and his Management Team. He explained the need to find out everything there was to know about the victim, particularly information concerning her movements during the 24 hours prior to the murder. He ordered his detectives to plague local informants in an effort to obtain more details that would assist. He informed those members of the press who stood on the periphery of the briefing that the police were in control and had a number of positive leads to follow up. He was confident that the Ripper would be caught sooner rather than later, but he knew that his words would only be a stopgap to partly satisfy the public for a short period of time. He desperately needed time and space to concentrate on the way ahead and focus all his energy and attention on what was now proving to be a nightmare investigation.

During the three-day period that followed the murder of Mary Kelly, everything suddenly seemed to stand still. The criticisms stopped, the constant badgering from the media stopped, and the demands from higher authorities were few. It was as though the whole of London was in a state of shock for the time being.

However, that was not the case with the Major Incident Room and Intelligence Cell. They became hives of activity as workloads increased dramatically. The following points were considered by Abberline and his Management Team:

1. As with the previous victims, Kelly was a known female prostitute.

2. For the first time the murderer had committed his crime inside premises.

3. There was no doubt that the scene was where the body had been found.

4. The victim was lying on her back in a similar position to the previous victims.

5. The victim's throat had been cut.

6. The victim's face had been mutilated.

7. Parts of the victim's clothing were neatly piled on a chair.

8. The violence used against Kelly was far more intensive than what the previous victims had been subjected to.

9. There was no apparent motive.

10. A fierce fire had burnt in the grate, and traces of women's clothing were found amongst the ashes.

Abberline turned his mind back to the possible reasons for the murders and the way in which they had been committed. The progression of violence used in the series supported a theory that the killer was 'playing to the audience', as though he needed to commit a crime that was more grotesque than any of his previous. Was this a method of increasing the horror and disgust felt by the police and public? A cry made for greater attention and recognition to those who, in his twisted mind, represented his enemies? The Senior Investigating Officer also appreciated that he was not looking for a normal person who thought like himself or other normal and sane people. That made any attempt to analyse the murderer's thought patterns more difficult, but Abberline considered the possibility of such a person having received past psychiatric treatment for the obvious mental disorder he suffered from. If that was the case, the next question to be asked was what caused such a mental disturbance in a human being that would result in the kind of carnage the killer had obviously taken pleasure in inflicting upon his victims?

Mary Jane Kelly – Areas to be examined

Abberline put the following questions to his Management Team:

1. What were the last movements of the victim? Could there have been a prearranged meeting with the killer?

2. Could a motive be identified from the degree of violence used against Mary Kelly?

3. Were there any witnesses who saw the murderer with his victim before walking her back to Miller Court?

4. What positive links were there to the previous murders?

1. What were the last movements of the victim? Could there have been a prearranged meeting with the killer?
It would appear from witness statements taken at the time that on the night of her death, Mary Jane Kelly was fairly desperate to obtain money. She was sighted in a number of local public houses accosting men, and appeared to be 'well intoxicated'. At about 11.45 p.m. Mary Ann Cox, a neighbour of Kelly's, saw her walk into number 13 Dorset Street accompanied by a short, stout man, who appeared to be shabbily dressed. The police failed to trace that particular man. Cox also stated that when she returned to Miller's Court at about 1.00 a.m. she saw that Kelly's light was still on, and she heard Mary Kelly singing inside her room. Cox was also a local prostitute, and stated that on the same night she left Miller's Court for a second time and returned at about 3.00 a.m. At that time, Kelly's room was in silent darkness. Cox then retired to bed herself and was awakened at 6.15 a.m. by a man's footsteps going out of Miller's Court, which she thought were a patrolling police officer's.

135

A witness, George Hutchinson, had been employed as a nightwatchman, and it would appear that, apart from the killer, he was the last person to see Mary Kelly alive. Hutchinson stated that he had seen the dead woman at about 2.00 a.m. in Commercial Street, which was off the Whitechapel Road. He knew Kelly fairly well, and both of them were regular customers at the same public houses. She had asked him for the loan of some money to pay for her rent, but he couldn't help her. Hutchinson was also destitute and was forced to wander the streets himself.

The former nightwatchman further stated that Kelly seemed to become distressed and walked away towards where another man was standing beneath a street lamp. He watched her stop and talk to the man. According to Hutchinson, they both laughed and then started to walk towards where he was standing. The man was holding Kelly around the waist. They walked towards Dorset Street and Hutchinson followed them from a distance. When he reached number 13 everything was in darkness, but he heard whispered voices coming from inside and assumed that Kelly was entertaining her client. Hutchinson then waited at the entrance to Miller's Court for approximately three-quarters of an hour before continuing on his way when he heard the footsteps of what he thought was a patrolling policeman walking towards him.

Hutchinson later gave to police officers an extremely detailed description of Kelly's client.

'About 5 feet 6 inches in height, 30 to 35 years of age, dark complexion, with bushy eyebrows and a thin moustache with twirled ends. He appeared to be well-to-do and was wearing a long coat trimmed with astrakhan, spats with light-coloured buttons, and a necktie that was fastened by a horseshoe pin. There was also a watch-chain with a seal and red stone.'

Hutchinson also stated that the man was carrying a small narrow parcel which was about 8 inches in length.

One other witness, Elizabeth Prater, a prostitute who resided in a room directly above Kelly's, stated that at about 3.30 a.m. she heard a female voice cry out, 'Murder'. It wasn't repeated, so Prater went back to sleep.

2. Could a motive be identified from the degree of violence used against Mary Kelly?

There were a number of options for the Senior Investigating Officer to consider. It was accepted that the killer must have suffered from a form of mental disorder because of the way in which he committed his crimes. However, he was also cunning in the way he moved around the Whitechapel area without detection, and could have been a local resident who went about his business without arousing suspicions. Whichever area the Ripper came from and whatever his motives were, he was obviously a person who had an extremely violent disposition that exploded upon killing each victim. The murderer could have been obsessed by a hatred of one particular prostitute or all prostitutes generally. His hatred could have been towards all females and he selected prostitutes because they were easy targets.

If the motive to kill was fuelled by a general hatred towards all women or just towards prostitutes, there must have been a reason for that. Either he had been the victim of a traumatic incident or terrible ordeal which had resulted in a major disturbance to his mental state, or he had witnessed an incident that had the same effect. Abberline and his Management Team would have sought advice from a highly qualified medical practitioner who possessed some expertise in psychiatric problems and mentally disordered persons.

If the killer was so unbalanced that he was a homicidal maniac who killed only for pleasure or self-gratification, then a motive

137

would not have existed. If, however, the killer's desires were fuelled by a sexual motive, then the situation would be clearer and enquiries could be aimed towards known sexual deviants. In the absence of a clear and confirmed motive, then all possible options should have been identified as major Lines of Enquiry by the Senior Investigating Officer.

3. Were there any witnesses who saw the murderer with his victim before walking her back to Miller's Court?

Apart from George Hutchinson, there were no other witnesses who physically saw Mary Jane Kelly in the company of a man. Police patrols had allegedly been increased and local vigilance committees had apparently decided to support the beat patrols. It is therefore surprising that the killer moved around the area without being seen, unless his mode of transport was by carriage. If that was the case, then he would have only remained on foot in a small area and for a short period of time.

The man seen by Hutchinson stood alone beneath a street lamp, as if waiting for a prostitute to pass by. It is possible that the Ripper remained hidden in the darkest shadows of a street before identifying his victim. Only then would he have to step out into the open, where it was necessary to converse and secure her confidence.

4. What positive links were there to the previous murders?

There were a number of factors present in the Kelly murder that were similar to the previous murders: the same area of Whitechapel hosted all of the Ripper murders, the way in which each victim was killed and the kind of violence used. Surprisingly, there does appear to have been insufficient attention given by the police to the increased levels of violence attributed to each case. It is difficult to imagine a more outrageous desecration of a human body than that of Mary Kelly's. In other words, with his last victim the Ripper reached a climax in the way he went about his work and in what he achieved. That fact should have been eventually linked with the knowledge that Kelly was the last victim of the series.

Could the killer have stopped his activities because he had now fulfilled his murderous desires, or because he was physically prevented by either imprisonment or death? The majority of unanswered questions relating to the Ripper murders lie within the small area in which he worked. To kill five women over a short period of time and within such a small area as Whitechapel, and avoid detection, are the remarkable facts that have mystified many observers since.

POLICE NOTICE.

TO THE OCCUPIER.

On the mornings of Friday, 31st August, Saturday 8th, and Sunday, 30th September, 1888, Women were murdered in or near Whitechapel, supposed by some one residing in the immediate neighbourhood. Should you know of any person to whom suspicion is attached, you are earnestly requested to communicate at once with the nearest Police Station.

Metropolitan Police Office,
30th September, 1888.

Printed by McCorquodale & Co. Limited, " The Armoury," Southwark.

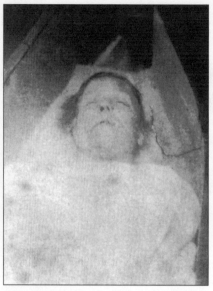

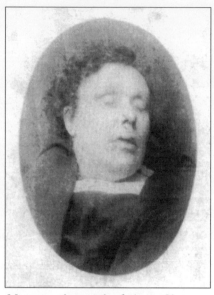

Mortuary photograph of Mary Ann Nichols,
Bucks Row, 31.8.88

Mortuary photograph of Annie Chapman,
Hanbury Street, 8.9.88

Mortuary photograph of Catharine Eddowes,
Mitre Square, 30.9.88

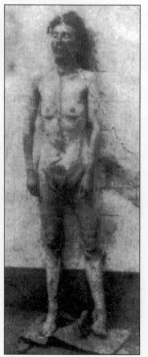

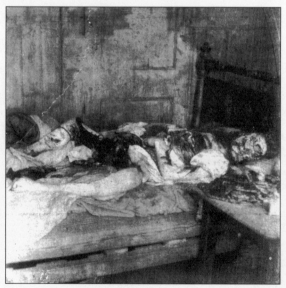

Mary Jane Kelly, Millers Court, 9.11.88

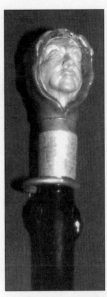

Face carved on the handle of a walking-stick presented to Frederick Abberline by his 'Ripper Investigation Team' upon his retirement

25. Sept. 1888.

Dear Boss.

I keep on hearing the police have caught me but they wont fix me just yet. I have laughed when they look so clever and talk about being on the right track. That joke about Leather Apron gave me real fits. I am down on whores and I shant quit ripping them till I do get buckled. Grand work the last job was. I gave the lady no time to squeal How can they catch me now. I love my work and want to start again. You will soon hear of me with my funny little games. I saved some of the proper red stuff in a ginger beer bottle over the last job to write with but it went thick like glue and I cant use it Red ink is fit enough I hope ha. ha. The next job I do I shall clip the ladys ears off and send to the police officers just for jolly wouldnt you. Keep this letter back till I do a bit more work then give it out straight My knife's so nice and sharp I want to get to work right away if I get a chance. Good luck.

yours truly
Jack the Ripper

Dont mind me giving the trade name.

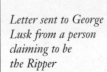

Letter sent to George Lusk from a person claiming to be the Ripper

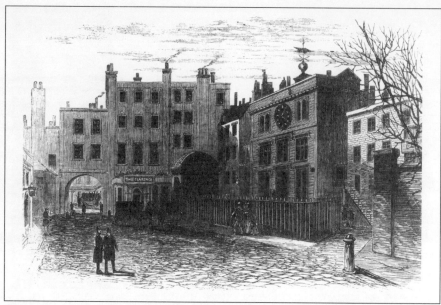

Sketch of Great Scotland Yard as it was during the Ripper murders until 1890

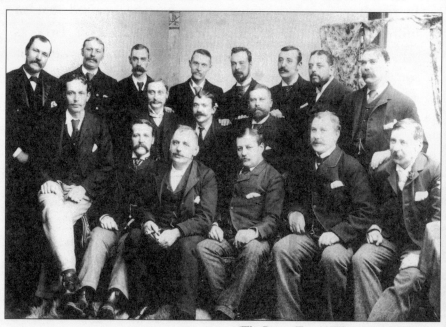

'The Ripper Team' (Whitechapel CID 1889)

Eight

The Senior Investigating Officer

The police officer given the responsibility of managing a major incident, such as a murder or series of murders, is normally referred to as the Senior Investigating Officer. Detective superintendents or detective chief inspectors are eligible for holding such positions, and the rank usually depends upon the circumstances and seriousness of the offence to be investigated. In recent years, many police forces have recognized that an individual's experience in criminal investigation isn't as important as the management skills he or she possesses. For some unexplained reason, it has always been difficult for a successful detective to develop into an achievable senior manager. The most effective Senior Investigating Officer should be a person who possesses a wide CID background together with some expertise in management skills.

Frederick George Abberline was a 45-year-old detective inspector at the time of the Ripper murders, who in reality was not the officer in overall command, but did lead the operational enquiries. Up until the early part of October 1888, the officer-in-charge was Detective Chief Inspector Donald Sutherland Swanson. He was later replaced by Doctor Robert Anderson, the assistant commissioner, Metropolitan Police CID, although Swanson continued to play an active role on the investigation. Anderson, who later received a knighthood, remained in command of the investigation until 1892.

Abberline had completed 14 years managing the Whitechapel Criminal Investigation Department, transferring to Scotland Yard in 1887. There is no doubt that he became a prominent figure in the Ripper enquiries because of his intimate knowledge of the East End and its criminals, in particular Whitechapel. His experience would be invaluable to a current similar investigation.

In today's police service, the old cavalier style of detective who relied upon strength of character and experience to drive major enquiries has long disappeared, with few exceptions. As a result of the quite dramatic increase in major investigations that has occurred since the early 1980s, the demands on police management have created a situation where experience in specialized fields is now a luxury. The required standards of professionalism and commitment throughout the senior ranks have also increased quite dramatically, as a result of new legislation and the development of higher management training and awareness.

Progress and further development in specialized areas of criminal investigation, such as forensic science and strategical planning, have also assisted in pushing supercilious attitudes into the background. Today's senior investigating officers are not necessarily better equipped with investigative skills, but are undoubtedly more knowledgeable about the managerial requirements laid down by the Home Office and Association of Chief Police Officers. The position requires a person who is more of a strategist and planner than his or her predecessors were using recognized management skills, supported by information technology.

The recent introduction of training programmes in subjects such as intelligence and interviewing techniques, has also given senior investigating officers access to better equipped and more professional detective officers and support staff. However, it is suggested that experience in the management of serious crime investigation is extremely valuable to any major enquiry and really comes into its own at the very beginning of an enquiry.

Adrenalin begins to rise when the telephone call is received during the early hours of the morning and the recipient is informed of a murder. The accomplished senior detective will immediately voice instructions to the person on the other end of the phone. In the majority of cases, he or she will request various personnel to attend either at the scene of the murder or somewhere close by. The officer will then have to drag himself out of bed, knowing that the next few hours will most probably be hard work, demanding and very stressful.

The less experienced officer might pause for a time whilst trying to mentally organize an initial strategy before listing the required priorities. It is acknowledged, however, that the majority of senior police officers, no matter how young in service, can make decisions instantly. Whether or not those decisions are made after assessing a situation accurately is sometimes the risk that is taken. They will usually arrive at the scene giving the impression that they are about to jump into a big black abyss, never to be seen again. It is suggested that such behaviour is normally overcome following words of advice and recommendation from an officer of lower rank but with more experience.

The majority of senior investigators do require a certain amount of credibility with those who have the responsibility of carrying out their instructions, and experience is usually the key to commencing a major enquiry on a strong footing and in the right direction.

The Management of Serious and Series Crimes Courses, held at the Police Staff College at Bramshill House in Hertfordshire, provide an opportunity for senior investigating officers from police forces throughout the country to meet and exchange views and ideas. The courses are designed for officers of the ranks of detective superintendent and detective chief inspector, who are likely to deal with major incidents in the future. A number of senior CID officers who have investigated major high-profile murder cases attend and lecture the courses. This enables the 'students' to develop their own skills further from the knowledge and experience shared by the visiting lecturers. Fred Abberline would not have had that opportunity in 1888. Also he would not have been able to rely upon the relationships between senior investigating officers that are cultivated during such courses, enabling individuals to contact each other for advice and consultation when dealing with complex cases.

Many police officers today would argue that the success of a major crime investigation is dependent upon the character, ability and skills of the Senior Investigating Officer. In many cases this could be true. The more prolonged and complex an investigation becomes, the more it might have to rely on the strengths and expertise of the man or woman leading it.

There are many pressures and stress-related issues that can create difficulties for the senior investigator, all coming from various sources. Demands from other senior officers or from the public through the press and media can, on occasions, have a detrimental effect on an investigator's effectiveness. However, the most common and potentially damaging cause of anxiety is often promoted internally, from within the structure of the investigation. Operational police officers and civilian support staff need strong and decisive leadership, particularly at times when enquiries become protracted and laborious. The majority of frustrations that occur during a Major Incident Enquiry can be overcome with the knowledge that the 'team' is working together, heading in the same direction and with the same objectives to be achieved, supported by the leadership or management. If confusion or pessimism exists at the top, it will

144

cascade down to those people responsible for completing the tasks responsible for the success or failure of the investigation.

There are two kinds of major investigation. The first is the one that is detected fairly quickly, as a result of sufficient evidence being present at the start of the enquiry to arrest and charge the person responsible for the murder. The other is the prolonged fact-finding operation, where there is little information to support the enquiries that follow the initial stages of the investigation. It is in the latter circumstances that the senior investigating officer is exposed to more criticism and unwelcome influence. It is then that strong leadership and management skills become a necessity.

There are basic structural and procedural guidelines for every senior investigating officer to follow. It is true to say that major investigations managed strictly within those guidelines can be detected successfully. However, in circumstances where an enquiry becomes high-profile and complex, such as the Ripper murders, increased pressure and stress are natural companions for the Officer-in-Charge. Unfortunately, if that officer is not capable of dealing with such problem areas, then personal careers are jeopardized. It is essential that optimism and professionalism are maintained throughout the duration of an investigation, and that usually will depend upon the style and methods used by the Senior Investigating Officer to conduct the enquiry. 'The proof of the pudding is in the eating', and when a police force is subjected to a major enquiry that attracts national interest, in the majority of cases the person with the most experience in the field of criminal management usually gets the job of managing that enquiry.

Fred Abberline would have felt isolated from other police officers on occasions during the Ripper investigations. Sometimes that would have been by his own design, and on others would be forced upon him by the position he held and the necessity to make unpopular decisions which every senior manager from all walks of life would be aware of. For a person to be placed underneath a microscope in today's environment, in which every move he or she makes and every decision taken, is analysed, evaluated and sometimes criticized, can be quite a challenging experience. Levels of stress for senior investigating officers can be reduced considerably by the strength of character of the individual officer and also by the amount of experience that person has in dealing with similar positions. What is clear is that there does not exist anywhere else in the police service a more stimulating and challenging role than that of a senior investigating officer.

Because of the increase in the number of murders committed today compared with previous years, only a few attract major national press coverage. Those that are plagued with the kinds of demands made by the public that existed in the case of Jack the Ripper, have become rare events. However, if a similar series of murders occurred today, there is little doubt that the Senior Investigating Officer would face the same pressures as did Fred Abberline and his Management Team in 1888. The major difference today would be a greater sharing of the management workload and decision-making process, than was the case a hundred years ago. Today other experienced senior investigators would be available to support and assist with such an investigation. The person leading the enquiry would have access to a wider range of experts than those available in Abberline's day, including a greater understanding and closer liaison with the press and media. The failure to detect a major crime would not be blamed on one individual or even a team of individuals. Public tolerance is much higher and perceptions greater, which promotes a better understanding and greater acceptability of the difficulties investigating officers are faced with.

Until recently it was a common feature of a major investigation for officers to work long and hard hours, including those responsible for directing and supervising the investigation. In most cases the result was poor performance and ineffectiveness, caused by fatigue and mental tiredness. There have been occasions when senior investigating officers have lasted days rather than weeks, before becoming too mentally and physically drained to continue. On a number of occasions senior investigators have been replaced because of their failure to command effectively, to the detriment of an enquiry. The most common problem for senior police officers to overcome is their own reluctance to accept that their performance is suffering as a result of too much commitment. In the majority of cases, officers do recognize the symptoms of stress and incoherency displayed by their senior officer, but the investigation continues 'below par' rather than any individual risking admonishment for trying to remedy the situation by advice and positive recommendation.

The professional and experienced Senior Investigating Officer today will assess the extent of the enquiry he or she has been given to manage, and work out a daily routine suitable to the circumstances and demands of that specific investigation. The stronger and more confident the leader is, the greater the levels of optimism will be amongst the operational crews responsible for the day-to-day enquiry work. Fred Abberline would not have enjoyed such freedom or comfort, but his ability to continue as the Senior Investigating Officer in the Ripper murders would not have been questioned or doubted by his own senior officers, therefore self-assessment would have been the only tool for him to use in trying to ensure that he conducted the investigations to the best of his ability. Furthermore, any mistakes made as a result of overwork or lack of concentration would only have been condemned without positive action being taken.

It has only been in more recent years that a need for effective communication between everyone attached to a major investigation has been recognized. Daily briefings between the management and operational officers are essential in promoting a general attitude of universal ownership of the enquiry for everyone involved. The need for police officers and support staff members to work together as one team is obvious, and it is the responsibility of the Senior Investigating Officer and Management Team to ensure that such a practice is maintained.

There is little doubt that Abberline would have confided in two or three other officers, leaving the remainder of the investigation teams unaware of how the enquiry was progressing or otherwise. The press and media would have been regarded as the enemy, and Abberline would have remained isolated from his operational officers. The majority of meetings attended by him would have been with his own senior officers.

Abberline's past experience and reputation as a good investigator would have earned him sufficient respect and credibility for his officers to have given him total commitment, no matter how distanced he would have appeared to them. Lesser experienced senior officers might well have had major problems in maintaining the same levels of commitment throughout the rank and file.

The Reviewing procedures of major cases are aimed towards making sure that there is sufficient support for the Senior Investigating Officer following the initial stages of an investigation. Before such a system was introduced, senior investigating officers would often seek advice from colleagues and recognized experts, whenever an enquiry met with difficulties. Such practices still continue, but a structured system of Reviewing can be helpful to a major investigation. Such a system would have been beneficial to the Ripper enquiry.

A successful senior investigating officer has to be a person of many trades. He or she should have the ability to think laterally and be able to deal with a number of issues or subjects spontaneously, at any given time. The SIO must also have the interpersonal skills to motivate large numbers of people as well as maintaining positive leadership. The capacity for managerial workload should be high, although the need to analyse and measure self-performance is also a necessity. The ability to plan and implement strategies, as well as communicate them to all personnel engaged on the investigation, is also an important requirement. To promote high work rates and enthusiasm, a senior investigating officer must constantly display total commitment to the enquiry with energy, drive and optimism. It is suggested from recorded comments made by members of the Ripper Investigation Team that Fred Abberline possessed all of those qualities.

Nine

The Management of a Murder Investigation

It wouldn't be everybody's favourite pastime to stand in a cold mortuary at 4.00 in the morning, watching a post mortem being performed on a murder victim. The pathologist calling you from a viewing point situated a fair distance away, to have a closer look at some interesting spectacle he or she had discovered, and then to discuss the significance of the finding in depth, isn't really everyone's cup of tea. It is suggested that many a senior investigating officer must have wondered at that time whether or not they were in the right job. Their thoughts could wander towards future retirement, away from such dramatic scenes and involvement.

In the majority of cases the post mortem signals the beginning of a murder investigation, and it is with that knowledge that a senior detective officer will dive into an investigation with priorities and requirements flashing through the mind. What do you do to preserve, collect and evaluate evidence? Important information and occasionally evidence can be obtained from a post mortem, but what happens to it? As with all other various pieces of intelligence thought to be of some value to the investigation, no matter how significant or otherwise, it is subjected to a process that will eventually place it into an appropriate category, similar to placing a piece of jig-saw into a part of the picture where it should comfortably fit.

151

The 'engine-room' that drives any major crime investigation today is the Major Incident Room or MIR. When in operation, the majority of MIRs are now supported by computer databases upon which information important to the investigation is recorded. The Lines of Enquiry, details of the scene, witnesses, suspects and many other nominated categories are all maintained by the computer system. For a senior investigating officer in charge of a major enquiry, the information technology that supports the investigation is invaluable and allows the senior detective to maintain an accurate picture of how the enquiry is progressing and what needs to be done.

Much of the work carried out by the police officers and civilian members of staff responsible for the maintainance of a Major Incident Room dictates the levels of efficiency and support an investigation team receives. The effectiveness of the way in which a major inquiry is conducted depends mainly upon the efficiency of those responsible for the daily running of the engine-room. The levels and intensity of training programmes provided for incident room staff are a deciding factor upon how adequate the staff are at fulfilling their responsibilities. Past experience of individual members is also a crucial factor which can influence the team spirit required, especially when pressures and demands begin to increase.

The structures of Major Incident Rooms are basically the same for every police force, no matter in which part of the country the investigation is conducted. The guidelines are national but the computer systems that support them are not, and there still exists incompatibility between some police forces and the databases they adopt.

An MIR is made up of different component parts, each having a different role to play, similar to the flight deck of an aircraft or the bridge of a ship. Members of staff are attached to individual sections with contrasting responsibilities, but in the majority of cases police officers and civilians are multi-skilled and capable of performing each other's role.

At the very beginning of an investigation, the first responsibility for a senior investigating officer is to open a Major Incident Room. This task should be completed even when instructions are being relayed to operational police officers to preserve the scene of the crime for examination. There is also the need to staff the MIR with the appropriate number of skilled people as soon as a murder is reported. The kind of skill areas required depend upon whether the room will be manual or computer-based, and that decision is usually taken very quickly and as a matter of urgency.

From the moment a murder or suspicious death comes to the notice of the police, a search commences for evidence, intelligence or information as to the circumstances and background to the case and the identity of the person or persons responsible. In most incidents there is a need to appeal for help from the public at the earliest opportunity, to trace witnesses and suspects. The workload that is generated from such requests for assistance and from the initial enquiries made, can become intensive during the first 48 hours of any major investigation. The consequential flow of information that comes into the investigation requires evaluation and recording. It is during these early stages that the Major Incident Room staff are required to work flat out in order to avoid an unmanageable backlog of material waiting to be inputted onto the computerized system.

It can be a regular occurrence for an incident room to fall behind during the first 24 hours or so following the start of a major investigation, as a result of the heavy workload experienced during the initial stages. Nothing can be more frustrating to a senior investigating officer than to have to wait for important information to be traced and made available to him. However, there are occasions when such backlogs cannot be avoided, particularly when operational officers have submitted numerous statements of evidence and other informative documents that need to be typed and then forwarded for inputting onto the system. It is during this period that the expertise and professionalism of the people manning the MIR is tested to the limit and the burden placed upon individuals' shoulders can become intolerable. It is also down to what happens during those first few hours that can decide how smoothly and efficiently an investigation will continue in the weeks ahead or until the guilty party has been identified.

The main link between the Major Incident Room and the Senior Investigating Officer is the Office Manager. He or she will be responsible for everything that appertains to the running of the MIR and that officer, who is usually a detective inspector or above, will be a member of the SIO's Management Team.

When identifying some of the problems that exist in the investigation of high-profile major crimes today, some sympathy and understanding can be spared for Fred Abberline and his staff, who were working without the facilities available today, and who were subjected to tremendous criticism. It is suggested that the 'electrically charged' atmosphere that is created during the early stages of present-day investigations would have been no less than in 1888. The first few days that followed each of the Ripper murders would have been chaotic and somewhat perplexed. Abberline would have been working with only a basic and rudimentary structure of an incident room, with few people, if any, given the task of recording what information came to the notice of the police. For the senior investigator today, the absence of the work environment and conditions in which investigators carry out their enquiries would be devastating. In addition, the support and operational facilities that now exist can make life a little easier for the SIO.

THE MANAGEMENT OF A MURDER INVESTIGATION

The success of any major investigation depends very much on the corporate approach and team spirit the Senior Investigating Officer is capable of promoting. The days when the senior detective had to depend completely on personal experience, character and skills have long gone, and the modern senior police officer now looks more towards the vast pool of resources available to be tapped.

The SIO should choose his or her Management Team carefully, bringing together a group of people who possess various skills necessary for managing the Lines of Enquiry chosen. There should exist amongst the members levels of expertise in areas such as scene examination, intelligence and information technology, in addition to the basic skills required to motivate and manage people.

The Senior Investigating Officer's own effectiveness in the overall running of the enquiry will rely heavily upon the efficiency of the Management Team. There should exist throughout an investigation a feeling of 'ownership' between every person involved, supported by individual pride and energy. Every senior member having a management role should be capable of working closely with those police officers and support staff members under their command. Daily briefings and 'two-way' discussions should be regarded as essential.

As previously identified, the principal objectives of a Major Incident Room include the accurate recording of information relevant to the crime being investigated and to show at any given time how many enquiries have been completed or still await completion. In addition an MIR can also assist in briefing officers who have been seconded to the operational side of the investigation at a late stage, by providing updated information relevant to management guidelines and directives and the current state of the enquiry.

The management of the MIR stops with the Office Manager. That officer is usually supported by a 'Receiver', whose job will be to collate all information and other material submitted into the incident room. A statement reader, usually of the rank of detective sergeant, will be given the responsibility of examining and evaluating every statement taken from witnesses. That officer will highlight pieces of information contained within a statement that warrant further investigation. Following that procedure, details are then passed on to an 'Action Allocator', whose job will be to record those details before being allocated to operational police officers for further enquiries to be made.

The majority of senior investigating officers usually require an administration officer responsible for general administrative work and the welfare of people engaged on the investigation. Other posts in a Major Incident Room include 'Indexers', who are tasked with recording information onto the computer system, typists, clerks and telephonists. The numbers of personnel required for each MIR will depend upon the nature and size of the investigation.

Two other roles that are fundamental to the majority of major investigations are those of the House to House Enquiries Supervisor and the Exhibits Officer. Both are usually police officers, either detective sergeants or constables who have received specific training in their respective roles. Teams of police officers allocated to the House to House Enquiries Supervisor will be furnished with a questionnaire which is standard across the country. Again, according to the circumstances of the investigation, questions can be added or deleted from the standardized format. Areas in which the house to house enquiries need to be completed are identified and geographical parameters initially set by the Senior Investigating Officer. They can be, and generally are, reviewed as the investigation continues. The Major Investigation Room records all details of the enquiries undertaken, and will show at any given time how many have been completed and the number of enquiries still to be expedited. Details of any possible witnesses traced during the house to house enquiries are initially recorded by the MIR and operational crews later tasked with interviewing those witnesses and obtaining full statements. It is absolutely essential that all enquiries made and 'actions' completed are recorded by the Major Incident Room. It is also widely accepted that, for whatever purpose, relevant information is not recorded, there will be an obvious failure to retrieve that same information if it is regarded as fundamental to the investigation at a later stage.

The role of the Exhibits Officer is extremely important in ensuring the security and continuity of articles of evidential value. In the majority of cases, the Exhibits Officer is given access to a secure room for the storage of exhibits and a room for maintaining the necessary records. Details of all exhibits are recorded on the MIR computerized system, although the majority of exhibits officers keep their own paper records that show movements of all items of property.

One hundred years on from the Victorian Ripper murders, one of the most difficult problems still facing the police service throughout Great Britain is the inability to make investigations in certain areas of the country compatible with each other. For instance where one force supports its major investigations with 'X' computer system, another force might well be using 'Y' computer system. When linked enquiries become necessary or an investigation in one force area crosses the geographical boundaries of others, then there is an obvious preference for the individual systems to be able to talk to each other. Each force will have its own investigative team, which will require access to information and intelligence available from all of the investigations that are linked. Unfortunately, compatibility of systems appears to have been overlooked in years gone by, and individual police forces have been allowed to adopt the system each one has thought is best suited for them. There was no central co-ordination to ensure that everybody was on line with each other. Where two separate forces join investigative hands to deal with the same enquiry and their MIR systems are not compatible with each other, then the outcome can be catastrophic, resulting in long delays and extreme financial burdens.

During the Stephanie Slater kidnapping inquiry, which was investigated by the West Midlands Police during the early part of 1992, problems were encountered when the decision was taken to link that investigation with the Julie Dart murder enquiry being conducted by the West Yorkshire Police. Both forces had different computer systems to support their investigations, neither of which were compatible with each other. Only one system could be used whilst the other was made redundant, following the transfer of all recorded data onto the system chosen to continue supporting both enquiries. The force that ended up with the unemployed hardware had to pay high rental charges for replacement equipment that was compatible with the other force's system. In addition, investigations were frozen for a period of three days, during which time information was downloaded and transferred onto the system chosen to continue. It is widely recognized by the Home Office and police service that there is a need for forces to introduce computer systems that are aligned with each other, and there is little doubt that the problems of today will be remedied in the future.

Historically the Metropolitan Police has always been the largest police force in Great Britain, funded by central government, with a commissioner in overall command and accountable to the Home Secretary. Before the amalgamations of forces which occurred mostly during the 1960s and 1970s, it was common practice for the 'Met' to provide a detective superintendent and a detective sergeant to assist with long-term high-profile investigations. With the exception of terrorist crimes and other specialized and organized areas of crime, such requests for assistance have now become rare.

Only in recent years, with the creation of other Metropolitan forces, has the majority of 'provincial forces' outside London had the capacity to investigate major crimes without the support of Scotland Yard.

In November 1980 Mr Lawrence Byford, Her Majesty's Inspector of Constabulary, commenced a review of the Peter Sutcliffe or 'Yorkshire Ripper' case at the request of the then Home Secretary, William Whitelaw. Mr Byford was assisted by an external advisory team, and one of his main objectives was to examine the conduct of that particular investigation. In January 1982 the Home Secretary made a statement to the House of Commons on the Byford Report that had been submitted upon completion of the Review. Amongst a number of criticisms made, the report referred to the '...*ineffectiveness of the Major Incident Room, which became overloaded with unprocessed information*'. The Home Secretary continued,

'...*with hindsight, it is now clear that if these errors and inefficiencies had not occurred Sutcliffe would have been identified as a prime suspect sooner than he was. Mr Byford's report concludes that there is little doubt that he should have been arrested earlier, on the facts associated with his various police interviews.*'

Byford's recommendations included addressing problems that existed with the management requirements of the investigation of a series of major crimes and the training of senior detectives and personnel working in Major Incident Rooms. Also found to be lacking was the command of investigations involving a number of crimes which crossed force boundaries. It was suggested that a need existed whereby the best detective and forensic science skills in the country should be harnessed to support major high-profile investigations together with computer technology.

159

There are now in existence national standardized administrative procedures which assist investigations involving more than one police force, but until all forces are supported by the same computerized systems difficulties will continue. Today a Senior Investigating Officer from one force can visit another and should feel at home with the procedures being practised, procedures that should duplicate those used by that officer's own force.

In 1888 fingerprints were not recognized as being important in the investigation of crime. The knowledge that no two people in the world have identical *minutiae* was not available. In other words, each person possesses different patterned loops, ridges and whorls on the underside of their fingers and thumbs. It was not until the turn of the century that such information was introduced into this country from Asia and was recognized as a major leap forward in criminal investigation.

The development of forensic science was almost non-existent. Blood, semen, hair and other human body tissues and fluids were not important. Only in the last ten years has Genetic Fingerprinting become widely recognized as a major weapon in the fight against crime. DNA Profiling is the breaking down of an individual genetic field and usually requires a minimum of eleven genetic bands for comparison purposes with other samples. If eleven bands identified from a sample of semen recovered at the scene of a Ripper murder matched with the same eleven bands taken from a suspect, then the field of forensic science would be called upon to support the fact that the sample taken from the victim belonged to the suspect. Scientists can state a fairly accurate number of odds upon which that suspect's DNA matches that found at the murder scene. If those odds are fairly strong, such as one in every million people in the population would have the same DNA, then the evidence can be quite conclusive.

In circumstances where a number of murders or major crimes had been committed by the same person, as with the Victorian Ripper murder cases, Byford recommended that an experienced forensic scientist should be attached to the Management Team. The role of the scientist would be to assist the Senior Investigating Officer with advice, liaison and co-ordination, and to act as an interface between the laboratories involved in the case investigations and the senior detective. In fact, many of the Forensic Science Laboratories today appoint certain members of staff to ensure that individual police forces are provided with an effective service similar to that recommended in the report.

During the Byford Review, relatives of murder victims were given the opportunity to make clear their own views on how the Yorkshire Ripper enquiry had been conducted. It was recognized that, in the majority of cases, the real victims of crimes are those that have been left behind: parents, wives and husbands, brothers and sisters. In recent years a great deal of emphasis has been placed on developing further the levels and quality of support given to victims of crime. In many serious crime investigations, police officers who have been trained in counselling techniques are given the responsibility of communicating with and supporting the families of murder victims. Close relationships with the officers are encouraged and usually extend to beyond the subsequent trial and conviction. It is widely accepted that from the punitive measures imposed upon the offender by the courts, the victim can obtain some therapeutic result that helps them to handle trauma more easily. However, it is suggested that that in itself is insufficient. Individually aggrieved persons need to be prepared for the traumas that are associated with high-profile investigations, whether resulting from media interest, people who cause distress although with good intentions, or from the trial of the accused. It has become a major part of a serious crime investigation to ensure that professional support is made available for those who need it.

In some instances the wives and other members of the immediate families of men convicted of murders have also been regarded as victims. They are some of the people who have been referred to as 'the hidden victims of crime'. Recognition of the need to support those people is far removed from the days when close relatives of individuals who had been responsible for committing high-profile crimes were also condemned with the convicted person.

The subject of Offender or Suspect Profiling is a fairly new area introduced to criminal investigation. It is based on the belief that the perpetrator of a crime usually leaves something at the scene which tells a story about himself or herself, for example, the levels of violence used against a victim, as in the Ripper murders, or the way in which violence was used either to gain control over the victim or that which results from a frenzied and excitable attack. Certain behavioural patterns can be linked with a series of crimes, as could be seen when examining each of the Ripper's murders.

Its origins come from the United States of America, where the Federal Bureau of Investigation has depended upon Offender Profiling since the 1950s. The first time such methods were recorded as being used in the United Kingdom was in the early 1980s, when the Metropolitan Police asked for the assistance of the FBI when investigating a serial rapist in the Notting Hill area of London.

The Leicestershire Constabulary used the expertise of a psychologist during the investigation of a serial killer responsible for the murders of two young girls. The same case was also the first in which DNA Profiling was introduced successfully. The DNA taken from samples left by the offender at the scene did not match that of a suspect who had been charged with the two murders. Subsequently he was released, and further enquiries traced the man who did have the same DNA Profile, who was later convicted.

Provided there is sufficient data for the psychologist to analyse, Offender Profiling can be of assistance to a senior investigating officer, not only as a benchmark for identifying the kind of person who has committed the crime, but also for supporting the interviewing officers who deal with the suspect following the arrest stage. It can provide an insight into what makes the individual respond to questions that target certain areas and add to the professional interviewer's armoury.

The future of serious and major crime investigation will depend greatly upon the further development of the information technology available. More professional under-standing of 'team development', forensic facilities and support, more structured use of the media, and more effective briefing systems will all help to improve the investigator's role.

Ten

The Missing Links

Policing by consent is more than just a concept in this country, it is the very foundation-stone upon which the police service is built. Since the first centrally organized police force patrolled the streets of inner London in 1829, police officers have had to adapt to the demands and requirements of the society they serve. Whether or not this accurately projects a mirror image of the customs and cultures that exist within various communities is debatable. In recent years, the yardstick by which the police service measures its performance is public opinion which it seeks and evaluates on a regular basis.

Legislation is an effective control source which decides on the levels of power and authority given to the police to administer the right and wrongs in society. However, the way in which that society reacts to police tactics and performance is also important. It is fairly accurate to say that 'the police service reflects the way in which society thinks'. Legislation is a tool used to ensure that police practices do, within reason, comply with the public's general requirements. Members of a police force are also members of the public and live within social communities, groups which are not restricted to police officers only, as is the case in other European countries.

The police service has always been a disciplined organization, reflecting the levels of discipline that have existed in all walks of life. In a highly disciplined society, the police service has, in the past, been greatly influenced by general social behaviour and acceptance of what is permissible and what is not. Prior to the late 1950s and 1960s, particularly before National Service was abolished, social habits and cultures were more rigid and regulatory. Members of police forces throughout Great Britain were also subjected to similar environments during their working days. In military fashion, each member was extremely rank-conscious, and there was little room for discussion or negotiation between the different tiers of responsibility. As society moved away from those ideals towards more liberal attitudes, so did the police service. Drastic and radical changes do not occur overnight, but slowly develop over a period of time.

The result of the social progress and development that first gained strength in the 1960s and early 1970s, is a multi-racial and multi-cultured society that is more receptive to the need for equality and equal opportunities than ever before. The demands for such social changes were also influential within the police service, and many far-reaching reforms have taken place in recent years.

Such required changes, which are driven by customer demand, produce improvement in areas of professionalism and organizational strengths. During the early to middle periods of this century, it is suggested that policing in this country remained rather stagnant. Although there have always been scientists willing to assist in criminal investigations, it was not until the late 1930s that the Home Office set up the first Forensic Laboratories. Detective Training Schools were introduced for the purposes of educating CID officers in investigative skills and awareness of current techniques and procedures. Today, officers undergo detailed training in many subjects of criminal law. These can include the investigation of sexual and violent offences, drugs, fraud, firearms offences, theft, evidence and procedures, and many other areas created and governed by legislation. They are also taught interviewing techniques and communication skills. In many cases the organization is driven by self-criticism and a belief that further improvement can be achieved, no matter how well current practices are doing.

The higher-ranking officers in the police service also complete senior management courses, dealing with subjects including the management of individual and team performances, team building, equal opportunities, interpersonal relations, and operational and strategic planning skills. Compared with the Victorian police service, today's police managers are far better equipped for dealing with major incidents or investigations.

Improvements in training programmes for detective officers have without doubt helped to increase the levels of individual professionalism, together with a more advanced and progressive service now provided to the public. However, the development of the Forensic Science Service must be the most highly recognized achievement to take place in recent years.

In many past cases in which forensic scientific skills have been used, powerful evidence has helped juries to convict or acquit many accused people. The scientist brings independent skills to support a criminal investigation. He or she will possess a tremendous amount of knowledge relevant to a specialized area of science. Such experts also have to be masters of sophisticated technology that exists for analysis and examination purposes. Today there are about 400 scientists in the Forensic Science Service, with a wealth of experience available to be tapped by senior investigating officers.

Forensic Science Laboratories have many varied roles to play when called to support a major crime investigation. For example, in circumstances where a firearm is discharged or an explosion created, there may be a requirement to mass-screen people for gunshot residues or explosive material, by taking handswabs. The pattern of bloodstains found at the scene of a murder, carefully investigated, could provide details of the nature of the attack on the victim and the type of weapon used. Traces of blood found on a potential murder weapon could be linked to a victim and, perhaps later, to a suspect.

In most crimes of violence there is physical contact between the attacker and victim. Scientists believe that every contact leaves a trace, and examination of clothing and other material things could result in the identification of valuable evidence. Contact traces include material such as textile fibres, soil or vegetation carried from one site to another by the attacker's shoe; impacted paint could be transferred to garments. In many cases, traces which cannot be seen by the naked eye are visible under the microscope.

Forensic biologists can provide valuable information from examination of a murder scene. Blood and other body fluids, fragments of skin, or nails belonging to the offender can be recovered and later compared with samples taken from suspects. Where a violent attack has been met with resistance, sample scrapings taken from beneath the victim's fingernails can sometimes reveal traces of skin or hair, or even perhaps blood, belonging to the offender. Intricate examination of hair can reveal whether it is human or otherwise, whether it fell out naturally, was pulled out or even crushed.

Until the late 1980s, conventional blood grouping offered useful information in eliminating suspects, but unless a rare group was involved, this seldom provided conclusive evidence. In 1988, one hundred years after the Ripper investigations in Whitechapel, the greatest scientific step forward in the investigation of violent and sexual crimes was made; DNA Profiling was developed from original academic research into one of the most significant discoveries in the field of criminal investigation since fingerprints. Doctor Jeffries conducted the initial laboratory research at the University of Leicester, and the potential of DNA Profiling is now widely recognized by both police and lawyers, and its use in criminal investigations has increased enormously in the past few years.

But what is DNA, or rather deoxyribonucleic acid? Forensic scientists tell us that the building blocks of any living organism are cells and there are multi-millions inside the human body. Inside every cell is a nucleus that contains chromosomes. Each chromosome contains the inheritance mechanisms and has a backbone of DNA. Each DNA strand is responsible for physical differences between individuals, such as sex, race, hair colour, height, and even susceptibility to disease. It is a genetic fingerprint or chemical blueprint which no two people have the same, with the exception of identical twins. The phrase 'DNA fingerprinting' has been commonly used by the media, but is inaccurate. DNA Profiling is what the service provides: a profile of a person.

The recent discoveries have not made conventional blood grouping obsolete. They are relatively quick and easy to perform, and at present, conventional grouping can, on occasions, give results in circumstances where DNA Profiling fails. For example, where the only samples available are from small or degraded bloodstains from which DNA may not provide very discriminating evidence. When a detective assesses the sizes of samples which scientists prefer, the following suggestions can be a strong guide for the investigator:

Dried blood on cotton approximately the size of a five-pence piece.
Dried semen on cotton approximately the size of a one-penny piece.

Provided samples have been stored in suitable conditions, i.e. frozen, they can last for years and still give a good result.

169

Semen is the most DNA enriched body fluid there is, but profiles can also be obtained from blood, saliva taken from the cheek cells, hair roots, muscle, organs and other tissues. The current method of DNA analysis does not work with saliva or skin. It can be used to compare a suspect's profile with a crime profile or one from another, earlier unsolved case. There have been instances when DNA has been obtained from blood samples kept from murder cases more than 20 years old and compared with present-day suspects. Convictions have resulted following positive comparisons being made. The development of DNA analysis and profiling can only progress and shorten the amount of time required for a result to be achieved. A national databank is now being created for recording individual DNA profiles of persons who are charged with serious criminal offences.

Other areas dealt with by the Forensic Science Service include glass identification, instrument marks, handwriting, footwear marks, suspicious fires, restoration of erased marks, metallurgy, and document examination.

In a series of murders similar to those committed by Jack the Ripper, if the Forensic Science Service had existed at that time with today's capabilities, scientists would undoubtedly have played a major role in scene examination. There would also have been a strong possibility that sufficient evidence to convict the person responsible, once identified, would have been available.

Criminal Intelligence is a fairly new concept that has been introduced into the investigative arena. It has always existed. The Victorian police officers had access to information provided by individuals who worked closely with, or were members of the criminal fraternity. Information was obtained from witnesses who helped police with their enquiries. The difference today is one of structural strategy. Whereby information can be valuable to an investigation, if it is subjected to a process of evaluation, then it can be recognized for what it is: either strong and reliable information, or weak, unreliable or useless.

There are a number of factors to be considered when analysing pieces of information: the reliability of the source from whence it came; the period of time that has elapsed between obtaining the information and acting upon it; whether it is historical or current; whether the quality of the information is sufficient to warrant further investigative or operational action being taken.

In a major investigation an Intelligence Cell can play an important role. Although all information is recorded in the Major Incident Room and subsequent actions are directed from there, the Intelligence Cell evaluates that information and can give support and direction to managers as to the number of operational officers that should be tasked with progressing enquiries relative to the information. If certain intelligence is thought to be of a low priority, then routine enquiries can be made. If, however, the need for high-prioritised action is recognized, then it should be subjected to more urgent attention.

Crime Pattern Analysis can also be an important tool to assist the senior officer investigating a number of murders committed by the same person. It is a process that develops and tests a number of inferences relative to criminal activities. In other words it identifies the who, what, where, why, when and how factors that are important in complex or extremely involved major investigations. With the help of information technology, crime analysis puts together bits and pieces of information to show a pattern or give a meaning to various occurrences.

From the information process charts can be created, each with different messages. For example, a number of crimes that include the *modus operandi* or methods used to commit each offence can be linked to each other, showing their association.

171

Sequence Charts can illustrate what happened, to whom, where and when. The following is an example of a basic Sequence Chart that could have assisted the Ripper Investigation Team to obtain a quick overview of the information available.

Elizabeth Stride Murder Investigation

11.45 p.m.	12.30 a.m.
West sees victim in Berner St. with man, 5'6", plump, middle-aged, dk clothing, peaked cap. 'You could say anything but your prayers.'	PC Smith sees victim with man of same desc. given by West.
	Witness Brown sees victim with same man.
11.30 p.m. 12 midnight	1.00 a.m.

Berner Street Sunday 30 September 1888

12.30 a.m.	12.55 a.m.
Witness Marshall stands in yard of club in Berner St. Nothing seen.	Diemschutz finds victim at scene.

They can include the last sightings of a victim prior to a murder, the times between which a murder occurred, details of individual witnesses, what they saw, where they were at the time, and any other useful information given to the investigating officers. They can be of valuable assistance when briefing police officers and are sometimes regarded as reference points to assist senior investigating officers, particularly in extended and prolonged enquiries.

Victim Profiles can assist in identifying common denominators that exist in each enquiry that could support a suggested motive.

172

Murder One

Victim:	Mary Ann Nichols
Known as:	Polly
Date of Birth:	1845
Age:	43 years
Place of Birth:	Whitechapel
Address:	No fixed abode
Description:	5'2", small delicate features, greying hair, high cheekbones with front teeth missing and a scar on her forehead
Employment:	Unemployed housemaid
Relatives:	Mother deceased. Whereabouts of father not known. Children – 3 sons and 2 daughters
Associates:	Ellen Holland and other common prostitutes from the Whitechapel area
Last seen alive:	11.30 p.m. Whitechapel Road, alone
	12.30 a.m. in Brick Lane, alone
	12.30 a.m. Thrawl St, alone
	2.30 a.m, in High St at Osborn St, alone
Time and date body found:	3.40 a.m. Fri. 31.8.88
Place found:	Buck's Row, Whitechapel
By whom:	Witnesses Cross and Paul
Nature of injuries:	Cut throat and multiple
Motive:	Not known at present

Murder Two

Victim:	Annie May Chapman
Known as:	Dark Annie
Date of Birth:	1841
Age:	47 years
Place of Birth:	Paddington
Address:	35 Dorset St, Whitechapel
Description:	5', stout build, dark wavy brown hair, blue eyes and thick nose, front teeth missing from lower jaw
Employment:	Unemployed street seller
Relatives:	Parents not known. Children – 1 daughter and 1 son
Associates:	Amelia Palmer, John Evans and prostitutes in the Whitechapel area
Last seen alive:	11.30 p.m. at 35 Dorset St, alone
	12.12 a.m. at 35 Dorset St, alone
	1.35 a.m. 35 Dorset St, alone
	5.00 a.m. Spitalfields Market, alone
	5.30 a.m. 29 Hanbury St with man – small and foreign
Time and date body found:	6.00 a.m. Sat. 8.9.88.
Place found:	Rear of 29 Hanbury St, Whitechapel
By whom:	Witness Davis
Nature of injuries:	Cut throat and multiple
Motive:	Not known at present

Murder Three

Victim:	Elizabeth Stride
Known as:	Long Liz
Date of Birth:	1843
Age:	45 years
Place of Birth:	Gothenburg, Sweden
Address:	32 Flower and Dean St, Whitechapel
Description:	5'5", dark brown curly hair, heavy boned but weak from starvation; all lower jaw teeth missing
Employment:	Unemployed domestic
Relatives:	Mother and father believed resident in Gothenburg, Sweden No children confirmed
Associates:	Michael Kidney, Elizabeth Tanner and prostitutes in Whitechapel
Last seen alive:	7.00 p.m. 32 Flower and Dean St, alone 11.00 p.m. Settles St, with smartly dressed man 11.45 p.m. Berner St with same man 12.30 a.m. Berner St with same man 12.45 a.m. Berner St with same man
Time and date body found:	1.00 a.m. Sun. 30.9.88
Place found:	Entrance yard to International Working Men's Club, Berner St, Whitechapel
By whom:	Witness Diemschutz
Nature of injuries:	Cut throat
Motive:	Not known at present

Murder Four

Victim:	Catharine Eddowes
Known as:	Many aliases, including Kelly
Date of Birth:	1842
Age:	46 years
Place of Birth:	Wolverhampton
Address:	52 Flower and Dean St
Description:	5'3", thin build, dark brown hair. Looks older than her age
Employment:	Unemployed hop-picker
Relatives:	Mother deceased. Whereabouts of father not known. Children – 2 sons and 1 daughter
Associates:	John Kelly and prostitutes in Whitechapel area
Last seen alive:	8.30 p.m. Aldgate High St alone 1.00 a.m. Bishopsgate Police Station alone 1.35 a.m. Duke's Place alone
Time and date body found:	1.45 a.m. Sun. 30.9.88
Place found:	Mitre Square, Whitechapel
By whom:	PC Watkins
Nature of injuries:	Cut throat and multiple
Motive:	Not known at present.

Murder Five

Victim:	Mary Jane Kelly
Known as:	Black Mary, Fair Emma, Ginger
Date of Birth:	1863
Age:	25 years
Place of Birth:	Limerick
Address:	13 Miller's Court, Dorset Street, Whitechapel
Description:	5'2", slim build, dark hair with attractive face
Employment:	Unemployed
Relatives:	Whereabouts of parents not known. Believed six or seven brothers and sisters, not confirmed. 3 months pregnant at time of murder
Associates:	Joe Barnett, Joseph Fleming and numerous prostitutes resident in Whitechapel
Last seen alive:	11.45 p.m. Dorset Street with man stout, shabbily dressed 2.00 a.m. Commercial St near Thrawl St with man 5'6", smartly dressed, 35 years, dark complexion with moustache
Time and date body found:	10.45 a.m. Fri. 9.11.88
Place found:	13 Miller's Court, Dorset St, Whitechapel
By whom:	Witness Bowyer
Nature of injuries:	Multiple and savage
Motive:	Not known at present

As can be seen, all of the victims were small in height and stature and, with the exception of Kelly, were all in their forties. Each of them was a common prostitute, and at the time of their deaths they all lived in the Whitechapel area. The specific days and times each murder was committed could also have been important when trying to establish a pattern to the killer's lifestyle. For example, the murders took place on either a Friday, Saturday or Sunday. Inferences could be drawn that the murderer was only 'available' between Friday evenings and Monday mornings. These factors could indicate that he was in full employment during weekdays. One other point of interest is that the earliest a victim was seen alive was at 12.45 a.m. in the case of Nichols. The latest time was 5.30 a.m, when Chapman was last seen alive. These periods of time would indicate that the murderer was free to commit his crimes at any time during the night of the weekends he did so. If he lived with a family that might have been difficult for him, unless he had reasons to be absent during weekends because of the nature of his employment, which is doubtful, or some other reason. It is more likely that he lived alone or in circumstances where his absence throughout a Friday, Saturday or Sunday night would not be noticed, or would be expected.

Strong relationships and close liaison between senior police officers and members of the Crown Prosecution Service can also assist a major investigation. It does not necessarily follow that lawyers should only become involved in criminal cases once a person has been arrested or charged with an offence. There can be occasions when there is a need for legal advice before deciding on methods used to collect evidence, even though a suspect has not yet been identified. For instance, if a police officer is to be used in an undercover or covert role, then the way in which that officer obtains intelligence that could later be used as evidence could make its later submission during a trial inadmissible if obtained outside the parameters of the law. An experienced senior investigating officer will obtain advice from the Crown Prosecution Service prior to an operation commencing. Although the CPS is an organization independent of the police service, it can offer valuable support, if requested, in the right circumstances.

There has also been a vast increase in the use of technology, some cases involving highly sophisticated equipment requiring high levels of authority for its use. Major improvements have been made in the fields of surveillance and covert policing, which again would have been invaluable to the investigation teams charged with identifying the person responsible for the Ripper murders. Closed-circuit television would undoubtedly have been made available in circumstances where the murders were being committed within such a restricted geographical area. The periods of time during which the crimes were committed would also assist in specifying when television or other surveillance would be used, for example, between 10.00 a.m. and 7.00 a.m. Training programmes for police officers involved in the craft of surveillance or the use of specialized equipment are intensive and time-consuming, but the results that are achieved by the skills developed can be in the majority of cases extremely rewarding.

The investigation of serious crime has also benefited from a number of other skill areas that didn't exist one hundred years ago. In 1888 murders were not such a common offence as is the case now, therefore the number of police officers who had the investigative and managerial experience of dealing with major enquiries were few. Today, there exist specialist squads of officers and support staff who deal with nothing else but major investigations. Their experience and knowledge contribute towards supporting teams capable of responding to assistance calls immediately and with confidence. Regional Crime Squads sited across the country work closely with each other and with individual police forces in dealing with major and serious crimes. The majority of forces have their own 'in-

179

house' crime squads that contain professional, highly dedicated officers who share a wealth of experience and ability between them. It could be argued that if there was a rapid decrease in the number of major crimes committed, the opportunities for investigative skill areas to develop and improve would also be limited. However, at present that seems highly unlikely, and if a serial killer similar to Jack the Ripper was committing a series of murders today, he would undoubtedly be challenged by a body of people who were vastly skilled and experienced in criminal investigation. They would also be supported by scientific and technological facilities that were highly regarded and successful.

Eleven

The Final Hypothesis

During the few days that immediately followed the horror of the Kelly murder, Abberline sensed a noticeable change in the attitudes of his Management Team and other personnel. At first, he believed his own powers of judgement had become distorted as a result of the trauma experienced from the last murder. He sat for about an hour in the Major Incident Room talking with staff and watching his people go about their business. He became a little confused by what he saw and heard, before realizing that possibly, for the first time since Annie Chapman had been murdered, everyone working on the investigation was performing with extreme deliberation and as one unit. The difference between now and before the Kelly murder was purposefulness. There was more resolution in the way officers and civilians were going about their duties and fulfilling their commitments, as though the murder of Mary Kelly had triggered something inside everybody that said, 'We must catch this animal at all cost.'

Conversations overheard in corridors and briefing rooms contained such phrases as 'This animal has to be caught', or 'This inhuman horror ... ', or 'This monster ... '. The practical jokes and light-heartedness that usually accompanied major investigations involving large numbers of people had disappeared. Every officer and civilian he spoke to answered him with serious tones in their voices and determined looks on their faces. There appeared to have been a general hardening of individual attitudes and determination, all aimed towards bringing the Ripper to justice. Action reports and enquiries had been investigated, checked and double-checked by the MIR staff to ensure that nothing had been missed. The intelligence staff had worked around the clock, researching known suspects and other crimes, seeking an association or link with the murders. Witnesses and local criminals had been made targets for surveillance, in the hope that they might unwittingly know the murderer and lead police officers to him.

Abberline thought to mention his observations to his Management Team, but then decided there was no point. He knew that his comments could be misinterpreted, and he didn't want to contribute anything that might dampen the enthusiasm that was being displayed by those working for him. What he constantly told his own senior officers was that the enquiry needed a 'break'; a piece of luck which would give everyone cause for optimism and thus strengthen the energy needed to continue accelerating the investigation forward. 'Be patient, we'll get there.'

Abberline did, however, experience a lot of personal disappointment and disillusionment, although he kept those feelings to himself. One of the major causes for concern was the obvious lack of professional information coming in from the streets. The majority of past enquiries he had been involved in had met with success because either he or another officer had received sound and reliable information from a professional informant or some other source. That had not been the case so far in the Ripper investigations, and he was puzzled and somewhat confused as to why. Informants had been tasked with searching the Whitechapel area for some lead or snippet of intelligence that might help to identify the murderer, but had failed to deliver anything of use to the enquiry.

On the fourth day after Mary Kelly's death, Abberline visited a local public house in Whitechapel Road, where he met one of his own trusted and reliable informants. The dirty, smelly and unkempt petty thief, whom the senior detective had known since his childhood, sat across the table looking down at the floor. He was only in his early twenties and had already served two periods of hard labour for larceny and brawling. Abberline placed a glass of ale in front of him. 'Robbie, what's happening, son? He couldn't just vanish into thin air; somebody must know who he is or what he is?'

'Honest, Mr Abberline, it's been as quiet as the grave. We don't think he's from round 'ere; he can't be. There's nobody who wouldn't do 'im in if they knew who 'e was.'

'You've never let me down before, son. Are we really trying hard enough? What about the toffs? Any toffs or spivs been seen around here lately?'

'No strangers. Honest, Mr Abberline, honest; if me own father was a blind beggar I'd shop him into yer for this one; honest, Mr Abberline.'

'What's the old gut feeling say then, Robbie? If he's not from around here, where then?'

'People are saying things, Mr Abberline. They're saying lots of things, but what they're really saying is that 'e don't just vanish into the blackness of night but holes up somewhere safe, yer know?'

'Away from here, Robbie, outside Whitechapel?'

'Look south, Mr Abberline. 'E aint from Kensington or Mayfair, Mr Abberline, that's fer sure. Look towards the river; that's what people are saying. The docks, guv; where else would 'e come from?'

'Keep in touch, Robbie my son, I'm depending on you.' That conversation cost the senior detective two more glasses of best ale and a florin for his informant.

Abberline left and decided to walk down Mansell Street towards East Smithfield and the London dockland. He made his way along Wapping High Street, and then stood for a while watching the steamers and commercial transporters loading and unloading. The docks were busy with men shouldering large sacks and boxes of cargo up and down the quayside. The majority of ships and smaller boats were either from foreign ports or were British Charters. He must have stood there alone for about an hour, hoping that some stimulating ideas or theories would come to him which would suddenly give him the answers to the real reasons why such carnage had taken place in such a short space of time. But alas, nothing. There was no sudden urge to instruct police officers to board ships and question members of the crews. In fact, Abberline felt more confused than ever before and decided to return back to his office at Scotland Yard. He even questioned the driver of the hansom cab he stopped to take him there.

'Guvnor, I gets loads of 'em coming off the docks at night. They just want a good time and to spend their dosh on 'aving one. We gets Chinks and Ruskies and Froggies and all sorts 'ere almost every night.'

When he arrived back at the Yard, evening was approaching quickly and Abberline's feet and hands felt in need of defrosting. The uniformed officer standing at the front of the building saluted him as he walked up the steps towards the great archway that gave access into the country's nerve-centre for criminal investigation. The senior officer acknowledged the other officer by tipping the front of his felt hat with his hand.

As he walked along the narrow, gas-lit corridor towards his office, he saw members of his Management Team standing outside. They stood in silence, facing him as he walked towards them, feeling cold, tired and hungry.

'Well, gents, what have we here?' Abberline unlocked his office door and beckoned everyone inside. Sitting back in his stout red leather chair, he placed his feet upon the oak desk. One of his detective chief inspectors, Matthew Thomas, was the first to break the news.

'We have him, boss; I do believe we have him. Forensic have just confirmed that semen has been recovered from Kelly's house.'

'She was a prostitute, where was it found?'

'On one of her aprons folded on the chair.'

'Fresh semen?' asked Abberline.

'None other than the killer's, according to Forensic, if not, then someone else who was present at the time of the murder.'

'DNA?'

'The DNA results will be through within three days.'

A wide grin appeared on Abberline's face, for the first time during the past five weeks. At last he had a motive; the killer had left his calling-card at Mary Kelly's. He was a sexual pervert, and the DNA Analysis would give Abberline a detailed portrait of the man who was now the scourge of Whitechapel. He felt excitement pour through his body to such an extent that his legs began to shake and he removed them off the top of the desk.

'Bless him,' said Abberline. The answer to his last question meant there had been sufficient semen for a DNA Profile. He couldn't believe his luck, but he knew that he would still have to identify the person to whom the DNA belonged. That particular task was easier said than done, but at least he would have the evidence to convict, once an arrest had been made. At least for now, however, his team of police officers had something to work on and work towards.

The following morning, which was the fifth day after Kelly's murder, Abberline received some further encouraging news. The crew of detectives who had earlier been given the job of investigating the shipping lines and traffic in dockland on the dates of the murders, asked to see him. He was handed the following information:

Date of Murder	Victim	No. of Ships Docked
31 August	Nichols	7
8 September	Chapman	18
30 September	Stride/Eddowes	12
9 November	Kelly	5

On each of the dates the murders had been committed, with the exception of the last date, 9 November, one ship had been present: the Russian-owned steamer, *St Petersburg*. She had entered St Katherine Docks on Wednesday, 29 August, and left on Sunday, 9 September, bound for Liverpool Docks. On Saturday 29 September, the same ship had returned and docked again at St Katherine Docks, leaving on Friday, 5 October, bound for Calais, France.

Further enquiries revealed that the ship carried a crew of 22 Russian and 5 Polish nationals. Lists were available at the Maritime Dockers Office in Wapping Lane. Abberline immediately directed that enquiries be made with the French police at Calais to trace the current whereabouts of the *St Petersburg* and further enquiries to confirm the country of origin and identity of the owners. In addition, the two detectives who had been completing the enquiries were supported by a further four crews made up of eight CID officers.

A briefing was called that afternoon, and groups of officers were tasked with revisiting backstreet lodging-houses, brothels, public houses and other such establishments. They were instructed to find out whether any person remembered seeing a foreign-speaking seaman acting suspiciously or behaving in any unusual way, anywhere in the Whitechapel area. Abberline emphasised the need to treat the enquiries as top priority and with urgency. He also told each officer that he did not want any information concerning those enquiries to be leaked to the press.

Following a conversation with Detective Chief Super-intendent Arnold, in which the senior officer was briefed on the developments of the past few hours, Abberline then requested that an application be made to the Russian Embassy in London for assistance in obtaining communication with the *St Petersburg* after the ship's details had become known. Arnold agreed and stated that he would seek the support of the Home Secretary.

Later the same day Abberline was informed that the Russian steamer had docked at Calais on Monday, 8 November, and left on the following Friday, 12 November, bound for the Ukraine. Lists of crew members had been faxed to Scotland Yard by the French police, but according to their list the number of ship's members added up to 21 Russian and 5 Polish nationals. One Russian crewman was not on board when the ship docked at Calais. The list received from the French was compared with the one recorded in London. The name of Andrea Chekensovsky was listed on the London document, but missing off the French list. Immigration were informed and asked for any details they were in possession of that were relevant to the missing seaman. The reply was received fairly quickly; there was no trace of an Andrea Chekensovsky on their files.

The following morning Detective Superintendent Abberline held a press conference at Scotland Yard and released the following statement:

'The Enquiry Team currently investigating the series of murders that has recently taken place in the Whitechapel area need to trace for elimination purposes the following Russian seaman:

ANDREA CHEKENSOVSKY

Chekensovsky was a crew member on the Russian steamer ship St Petersburg *which has recently visited St Katherine Docks, London. Officers wish to speak to Mr Chekensovsky as a matter of urgency, and believe he may still be living in the London area. Any person having any knowledge of the whereabouts of this man should telephone the Murder Incident Room or contact their local police station.'*

Abberline then left the deluge of press enquiries and reporters' questions to the Force Press Liaison Officer, Betty McGuire.

During that evening, the Senior Investigating Officer met with Arnold and was advised to progress this particular line of enquiry with some caution. 'We don't want to start a hue and cry for every foreign seaman visiting London, Fred, now do we?'

Abberline supported his suspicions with the boot prints that had been found at the scenes of the first two murders, which were similar to those worn by seamen, and the fact that the *St Petersburg* was present in London Docks at the same time the murders were committed. He also pointed out that once he got his hands on Chekensovsky, he could verify his innocence or guilt by comparing his DNA with that recovered from the Kelly scene, which was still being analysed.

'What about the last date, when Kelly died, Fred? The *St Petersburg* wasn't around then. Can you explain that yet?'

'No, but I'll know more about that once we have contacted the ship's captain.'

'The Home Secretary is naturally concerned that we should avoid an international incident, Fred, you know what it's like. We have to tread carefully. There is a possibility we could lock up the wrong man, and then there would be hell to pay.'

188

'For Christ's sake, Tom, the man has butchered five prostitutes and all of London is screaming for our heads, and rightly so; and you're bothered about a bloody Home Secretary that's frightened of his own bloody shadow. I don't give a shit about whether or not this will cause an international incident, Tom, I'm going to lock the bastard up.'

Arnold didn't pursue his arguments further and thought it best to allow the veins in Abberline's neck, which had expanded quite considerably, an opportunity to subside.

The following two days were extremely frustrating for Abberline because of a lack of progress in contacting the *St Petersburg*. Eventually the Russian Embassy faxed the following statement to the Foreign Office, who passed it to Scotland Yard.

'First Class Seaman Andrea Chekensovsky was a member of the St Petersburg's *crew until Thursday, 4 October 1888, when he was paid up in full, having decided to transfer his registration to the Russian steamship* Katrina *due to return to a Russian port in November. Seaman Chekensovsky is a Russian citizen who has now attained his 28th birthday. Captain Petrovich describes him as being 5'6" tall, medium build with dark brown hair cut short, thin face with pointed features and a moustache. Chekensovsky is believed to speak a little English. He has informed Captain Petrovich that his intentions are to return home to Russia aboard the* Katrina.'

Further enquiries revealed that the *Katrina* had docked in London Docks on Monday, 1 October 1888, and had left on Monday, 8 October, for Newcastle. The same steamer had returned to London Docks on Wednesday, 7 November, and left on Saturday, 10 November, bound for Russia with a cargo of heavy machinery.

189

Abberline immediately requested the help of the Russian Embassy to arrange for the arrest of Chekensovsky as soon as possible and for deportation procedures back to the United Kingdom to commence. Unfortunately there was no Extra-dition Treaty between Russia and the United Kingdom, but the Russian Embassy officials promised the Scotland Yard detective that they would do everything in their power to assist.

Mary Jane Kelly was the last victim of the serial killer known as Jack the Ripper, and although Abberline's investigation team continued searching for further clues as to the killer's identity, very little further information was forthcoming during the three-month period that followed Kelly's murder. Eventually, all of the forensic results were received by the Major Incident Room. When examining the major points upon which forensic evidence would be given in a future trial, Abberline was optimistic. All he needed was the man who could match the following identified factors:

1. The size 8 boot prints recovered from the murder scenes of Nichols and Chapman.

2. The recovered woollen fibres containing blackberry dye.

3. Blood samples taken from the piece of apron belonging to Catharine Eddowes, recovered in Goulston Street, had been identified as belonging to the victim.

4. Some of the bloodstains recovered from the public wash-basin in Dorset Street near to the Eddowes murder scene, had been identified as belonging to the victim; however, there were other samples recovered which had not come from Eddowes. There were sufficient 'foreign' samples to complete a DNA Profile.

5. The semen stains recovered from the murder scene of Mary Kelly had been sufficient for DNA Analysis. These matched with the blood samples taken from the wash-basin in Dorset Street.

Abberline urgently needed a blood sample from the Russian seaman who had now become the main suspect.

It was a bright sunny spring morning when the Senior Investigating Officer stepped from his carriage outside the front steps of Scotland Yard. He looked skywards and could not see a cloud in sight, although there was a slight breeze that carried a sharp warning of winter not having totally disappeared.

A cup of hot coffee gave Abberline sufficient comfort and stimulus on which to start the day's work. He was still trying to imagine the seaman's facial looks, which hadn't really left his mind for the past three months, when there was a knock on the door. It was Albert Davey, Abberline's detective chief inspector responsible for operations.

'At about eleven o'clock last night, PC Watkins, who found Catharine Eddowes' body, stopped a man in East Smithfield who told him that he was working as a loader in St Katherine Docks. He spoke with a foreign accent and gave his name as Yuri Igonov from the Ukraine. He didn't have any documents or other identification on him, and apparently looked the suspicious type. Anyway, Watkins took him into Bishopsgate, where he is now. He's so far given two addresses which have proved to be false, and some of the lads are round at another one in Cavell Street, Whitechapel, at the moment.'

Abberline asked, 'What does the suspicious type look like, Bert?'

'Well, apparently he was just evasive and Watkins didn't like the look of him.'

'Did he have anything with him?'

'Not as far as I know, but I've only just been told about it.'

191

'Do we know what he was wearing?'

'No, but I'll find out. By the way, apparently he answers the same description as Chekensovsky.'

'Keep me informed, Bert.'

The Detective Chief Inspector left to obtain more information.

Andrea Chekensovsky had failed to board the *Katrina* after leaving the *St Petersburg* on 4 October 1888. Instead, he had worked as a casual seaman on a British steamer which he left when the ship docked in Liverpool towards the end of November. He had then worked at a number of jobs in Liverpool before eventually returning to London on the day before PC Watkins had arrested him.

Number 23 Cavell Street was a typical backstreet lodging-house in which rooms were let for fourpence a night by the landlord, Michael Straw. When police officers spoke to Straw, he told them that the Russian had arrived the day before and paid him two shillings and fourpence, being a week's rent in advance. The new lodger was given a room at the very top of the house, in the attic, after he had apparently declined the offer of a room on the first floor. When his room was searched by police officers, they found the following items before requesting the support of a scenes of crime team:

One black woollen cloak.

Two pairs of woollen trousers, one black and one brown.

Three shirts, two heavily patterned, and one plain white shirt.

One detached white shirt collar.

One pair of black leather boots, the soles of which had deep ridges scored across them.

Three small ladies' handkerchiefs, one of which appeared to be bloodstained.

A large number of newspapers and journals dated between 31 August and 1st October 1888, all carrying stories about the Ripper murders.

In addition, there were a number of private papers which were mostly written in Russian, and a number of sketches of the Whitechapel district with various sites marked by circles. Those included Bucks Row and the Jews' cemetery, Hanbury Street, Mitre Square and Dorset Street, all scenes of the Ripper murders. Surprisingly, there was no circle or other mark around Berner Street, the scene of Elizabeth Stride's murder.

Detective Superintendent Abberline was informed within minutes of the discovery, and immediately punched the air with a fist. He felt all the frustration of months of anguish and torment leave him. His initial reaction was accompanied by heavy exhaling to the sound of a loud 'Yeeees'.

The room which had been rented by the suspect was treated as another murder scene. Arrangements were made for photographs to be taken before anything was disturbed. Abberline then asked for a team of forensic scientists to search and recover any article likely to be of evidential value and requiring laboratory analysis. Both the scientists and police officers carefully and individually packaged every article thought to be of significance, and those requiring forensic examination were transferred to the laboratory. Other items were taken by exhibits officers to the Major Incident Room. Details of every object seized would be given to the incident room staff for inputting onto the computer.

Experts worked constantly through that day and the following night, meticulously examining all parts of the room, including above and below the floorboards. Even the walls and ceiling of the room that had now become the focal point for both police and the world's press, were examined for bloodstains, fingerprints and any other impression or material that could assist the investigation.

All the comings and goings to and from the house in Cavell Street were recorded by a barrage of television cameras that had taken up residence on the pavement opposite number 23. Barriers were set up and manned by uniformed police officers to remind the members of the media that a boundary line did exist and they were not to cross it. The Senior Investigating Officer had already issued an order that no interviews were to be given to the press. It was Abberline's intention to release a statement once most of the facts were known, and he was aware that anything said before or after any charges had been preferred could be regarded as being sub-judicial to the case at a later trial.

Within the hour of learning about the developments in Cavell Street, both Arnold and Abberline were walking into Bishopsgate Street Police Station, which had become a hive of activity. Even before the two senior officers had entered a ground-floor office which had been designated for them, journalists were in attendance in the front office, shouting for comments from Abberline. The Senior Investigating Officer walked up to the group of reporters, smiled broadly and walked away in silence.

Twelve

An Audience with Jack the Ripper

One of the principal strengths of a CID officer has always been the ability to interview suspects for crime and successfully extract information from them, whether or not guilt or innocence is indicated as a result of the interview. Only since the mid-1980s have police forces introduced structured interviewing development courses that make officers aware of a number of aspects of a suspect's behaviour that can assist in assessing whether or not that person is telling the truth or lies. Completion of such training programmes, together with experience of live interviews, can produce a professional interviewer who possesses strong interrogative skills.

In 1888 interviewing police officers would have been dependent upon their own intuitions or 'gut feelings' as to whether or not a person was guilty of an offence. In the majority of cases, such premonitions would have been based on experience gained from observing how older and more established detectives performed and copying what they had seen and learnt.

The following is a fictionalized account of an interview that could have taken place between Detective Superintendent Abberline and the person responsible for the Whitechapel murders. If such an interview were to take place today, there are a number of legal requirements that would have to be observed. The suspect would be given access to a solicitor and the opportunity to discuss his position in private with his legal representative prior to an interview with police officers. Any subsequent interview would be recorded on videotape, provided the suspect agreed. If not, audio recording equipment would be used. The suspect's solicitor or legal representative would then be invited to remain throughout the interview and advise his client as to what answers he should give to the questions put to him. The following interview takes into consideration the fact that in 1888 no such rights would have been available to a suspect arrested for a crime.

The answers put to the suspect have been based on a psychological profile of Jack the Ripper prepared by a leading psychologist and crime analyst who is currently a member of the police service. The actual profile follows the interview.

Abberline was accompanied by Arnold when both men entered the interview room. The suspect sat in a chair facing the door. The only other furniture in the bare room were two chairs and a desk that was situated between the interviewing officers and the suspect.

The senior detectives sat and faced the suspect. Abberline commenced the interview with the intention of developing a little rapport with the suspect, aimed towards promoting a two-way conversation between them.

Abberline:	'Do you speak English?'
Suspect:	'A little.'
Abberline:	'Can you understand what I am saying to you?'
Suspect:	'Yes.'
Abberline:	'What is your native language?'
Suspect:	'Russian, I speak Russian.'

Abberline:	'Would you like me to get a Russian interpreter for you?'
Suspect:	'No.'
Abberline:	'Very well. I understand that you have given your name as Yuri Igonov. Is that correct?'
Suspect:	'Yes.'
Abberline:	'Is that your proper name?'

There was no reply.

Abberline:	'Is Yuri Igonov your correct name?'
Suspect:	'No.'
Abberline:	'Would you like to tell us what your real name is then?'

There was no reply.

Abberline:	'Is your real name Andrea Chekensovsky?'

The suspect slowly raised his eyes from the table in front of him and replied, 'Yes.'

Abberline remained silent for a while and stared into Chekensovsky's eyes. He saw nothing, only coldness. There were no messages to be read from the way in which the Russian stared back. His gaze did not disclose any signs of feelings or fear, only a vacant look. Chekensovsky then lowered his eyes back to the table.

Abberline:	'Do you know why you are here?'
Chekensovsky:	'Yes.'
Abberline:	'Tell me why you think you are here.'
Chekensovsky:	'Because you think I killed those women.'

The interview was interrupted by a loud knock on the door that caused all three men to turn to see who and what it was. Detective Chief Inspector Davey opened the door. 'Sorry, guv, can I have a quick word outside? It's important.'

Abberline left the room and stood outside with Davey in the corridor.

'I think we've got the knife. It was in a bag found in the room. I understand it was wrapped in some newspaper. Forensic have whipped it off to the laboratory.'

'What's it look like, Albert?'

'According to the scenes of crime kid, it's got an eight-inch blade about half an inch wide. It's very sharp and goes down to a point at the end. He described it like a butcher's filleting knife.'

Abberline returned to the interview room and sat down and stared at Chekensovsky, who was still looking down at the table top.

Abberline: 'Do you own a knife, Mr Chekensovsky, about eight inches in length and half an inch wide?'

The police officer asked the question with a smile on his face, inviting both the suspect and Arnold to look at him, which they did, Arnold showing more surprise than the Russian.

Chekensovsky didn't reply.

Abberline: 'Tell me again, Mr Chekensovsky, why you think you are here.'

Chekensovsky: 'Because of the women I have killed.'

Abberline looked directly across towards Arnold, who coughed to clear his throat.

Abberline: 'Go on, tell us more.'

Chekensovsky: 'Ask me the questions. I will tell you what you want to know.'

Abberline: 'How many women have you murdered?'

Chekensovsky: 'Four or five here.'

Abberline: 'Four or five here. How many more elsewhere?'

Chekensovsky: 'Only four or five here.'

Abberline: 'Then let's just talk about the four or five women that you have murdered here. Were they any particular type of woman?'

Chekensovsky: 'Prostitutes.'

Abberline: 'How did you select each of your victims? Did you know them beforehand and then just waited to follow them before committing each murder?'

Chekensovsky: 'No that's not true. I didn't know any of them, except...'

Abberline: 'Go on.'

Chekensovsky: 'I think I might have met the last one or seen her somewhere before.'

Abberline: 'You mean Mary Jane Kelly?'

Chekensovsky: 'I didn't know her name; the one in the house.'

Abberline: 'Where had you seen her before?'

Chekensovsky: 'I'm not sure. Perhaps in a corner house.'

Abberline: 'You mean in a pub?'

Chekensovsky: 'Yes, in a pub, but I didn't know any of them. I just walked the streets looking for a victim, and when I saw one I talked to them and it used to happen.'

Abberline: 'I know that the answer to this question might seem obvious, but why did you attack your victims at night?'

Chekensovsky: 'Because I felt comfortable in the darkness.'

Abberline: 'Are you very familiar with the Whitechapel area?'

Chekensovsky: 'Yes, I know it well. I have spent a lot of time here in the past.'

Abberline: 'What made you murder five prostitutes?'

Chekensovsky: 'A mixture of sexual fantasy and anger. When I did the first murder, the fantasy became reality and I got excitement from what I did. Afterwards I felt some guilt, but that soon went away and I moved on to the next woman to get the same excitement as before.'

Abberline: 'Have you ever been involved in any ritualistic practices during your past life?'

Chekensovsky: 'No, never.'

Abberline: 'Then how do you explain some of the horrendous things you did to your victims, including the neat piles of internal organs and items of property belonging to them?'

Chekensovsky: 'I got the same excitement from doing that as when I committed the murders and butchered them.'

Abberline: 'So what you are saying is that you achieved the same excitement from displaying your work in such a macabre way, as you did when you cut their throats?'

Chekensovsky: 'Yes, but in a way the excitement was continuous.'

Abberline: 'So you were dominated by your fantasies and ritualistic actions?'

Chekensovsky: 'I don't know; yes.'

Abberline:	'Did you always keep the knife you used with you before and after each of the murders?'
Chekensovsky:	'Yes, it was the tool of my trade. I always carried it wrapped up in newspaper or something the same. That is the one you have obviously found.'
Abberline:	'How were you dressed at the time of each murder? Did you always wear the same clothing?'
Chekensovsky:	'I was always smartly dressed.'
Abberline:	'Why?'
Chekensovsky:	'Because I knew that no one would challenge me or stop me if they thought I was a gentleman of substance. In most cases I wore the same clothes, yes.'
Abberline:	'Have you ever been professionally employed?'
Chekensovsky:	'No, but I was a carpenter before I went to sea.'
Abberline:	'Do you have much of a social life?'
Chekensovsky:	'Yes, when I feel like drinking I drink, and I like to mix with the people.'
Abberline:	'Do you drink much alcohol or use any drugs?'
Chekensovsky:	'I have never used drugs, and I would say that I am a moderate drinker of alcohol.'
Abberline:	'Had you drunk any alcohol before you committed any of the murders?'
Chekensovsky:	'No, I don't think so.'
Abberline:	'So drink wasn't the cause of your actions when you killed those women?'
Chekensovsky:	'No, I cannot use that as an excuse.'

Abberline: 'Can you remember what you did to your victims and how you felt at the time?'

Chekensovsky: 'Yes, I can, and I enjoyed what I did at the time. They were things that I didn't feel I had to do; I wanted to do them.'

Abberline looked towards Arnold with a look of disgust in his eyes, and his senior officer continued to stare at the suspect, expressionless.

Abberline: 'You said earlier that your motives were both sexual and anger. Was there something that happened to you in the past that caused you to feel the way you do?'

Chekensovsky: 'I do not want to talk about my past. I have been treated like dirt by many women, for a number of reasons, but I do not want to talk about them.'

Abberline: 'Had you ever been with a prostitute sexually before you started committing the murders?'

Chekensovsky: 'Yes, but I do not wish to talk about it.'

Abberline: 'How did you used to get on with your parents during your childhood?'

Chekensovsky: 'I didn't know who my father was, and lived with my mother. She used to have men friends call at the house and take them into the room at the back. I used to hear bad sounds that used to depress me.'

Abberline: 'What kind of bad sounds?'

Chekensovsky: 'Sometimes she would be laughing and other times she would scream. I used to sit in the dark, looking at the light from the next room that shone between the cracks in the door.

Voices were muffled, and I used to cry and felt very alone.'

Abberline: 'Was your mother a prostitute?'

Chekensovsky: 'I've told you, I don't want to talk about that any more.'

Abberline: 'When you said that you used to converse with your victims, in what way? What did you say to them?'

Chekensovsky: 'I used to charm them and then offer them some business.'

Abberline: 'Did you ever feel the desire to control them, you know, control them completely?'

Chekensovsky: 'Always. They had to be silenced so they couldn't resist me. I enjoyed being the master of them. They couldn't hit back, and it gave me more time to do what I wanted to do.'

Abberline: 'So what did you want to do to them?'

Chekensovsky: 'Master them. I wanted to show everybody that I could master these women.'

Abberline: 'So that's why you cut them up, is it?'

Chekensovsky just nodded his head.

Abberline: 'So you knew exactly what you were doing to them at all times?'

Chekensovsky again nodded.

Abberline: 'Did you think that they all looked similar in appearance?'

Chekensovsky: 'They were all prostitutes.'

Abberline: 'Yes, but I mean physically and facially. Did they all look the same to you?'

Chekensovsky: 'I think so, yes.'

Abberline: 'Did they remind you of someone else?'

Chekensovsky: 'I don't wish to talk about that.'

Abberline: 'Did you look for victims that had a certain appearance?'

Chekensovsky: 'I don't understand. I might have done. I think I did, yes, they all looked the same.'

Abberline: 'Did any of them look like your mother?'

Chekensovsky did not answer and just looked into Abberline's eyes.

Abberline: 'Were there any other women you accosted but didn't murder?'

Chekensovsky: 'A few.'

Abberline: 'Why didn't you murder them?'

Chekensovsky: 'Because they didn't look right, and on one occasion there were too many people about and she wouldn't come with me.'

Abberline: 'So there was a particular person who you sought to kill; one who looked and dressed in a specific manner?'

Chekensovsky: 'I suppose so, yes.'

Abberline: 'The victims in your last two murders, Catharine Eddowes and Mary Kelly, had their faces partially mutilated. Can you explain why you did that to those two women and not the others?'

Chekensovsky: 'Because I didn't want to look at their faces. They reminded me of something horrible so I removed their looks.'

Abberline: 'Was that someone else your mother?'

Chekensovsky: 'No; I don't want to talk about that any more.'

Abberline:	'On Sunday, 30 September 1888, you murdered a prostitute by the name of Elizabeth Stride in Berner Street. You then murdered a second prostitute, Catharine Eddowes, in Mitre Square on the same night. Can you tell me why you killed the second woman having already murdered once that night?'
Chekensovsky:	'Because I was angry. I couldn't finish the job with the first one because somebody came, so I walked back towards the docks when I bumped into the second girl, and you know the rest.'
Abberline:	'You had no fear of being caught?'
Chekensovsky:	'My desires were too great; I never considered being caught. I had to do what I did to quench my thirst.'

Abberline stood up and again left the room. He returned after a short while and placed a pot of ink and pen on top of the table. He then pulled a piece of paper from out of his inside pocket and also placed that on the table in front of Chekensovsky.

Abberline:	'Mr Chekensovsky, I want you to write your full name in English, on this piece of paper.'

Chekensovsky picked up the pen with his left hand and did what he had been instructed to do. Abberline smiled and picked up the piece of paper, looking at Arnold.

'Left-handed, Tom. Thank you, Mr Chekensovsky.'

Both officers then left the room and the interview was concluded.

Psychological Profile of the Man Known as 'Jack the Ripper'

The following analysis has been based on the material made available from the initial investigation into the Whitechapel murders committed in 1888. A number of comparisons have been made with other known serial killers both in the United States of America and Great Britain.

The motive behind each of the murders is primarily a sexual one. That, together with ritualistic elements, would dominate the killer's intentions. This is supported by a number of factors, including the nature of some of the injuries inflicted to the genitals and around the necks of the victims. Any attack or assault on the region of a female's neck can be interpreted as sexual. The purpose behind such acts as the neat piles of items left at the scenes of some of his crimes and the placing of internal organs on top of his victim's bodies would be to display his work, although he did not leave any real evidence behind.

There also exists an element of precipitating situational stress, where the person has a fantasy which is realized when he commits the first murder. This is then followed by a period of guilt, although the presence of such a state of mind in these cases is doubtful. The fantasy is then re-enforced and the cycle continues with the commission of the second and additional murders.

None of the victims were subjected to blitz attacks. From some of the evidence obtained from witnesses, it would appear more likely that there was some degree of interaction prior to each attack.

Psychosis would be the most likely element to drive the killer towards achieving his objectives, rather than the use of drugs or alcohol. His predisposition would most likely be caused by events in the past that caused the killer personal psychological disturbances and anguish, such as being laughed at or ridiculed by a woman or women over a period of time. There is a likelihood that the victim would be targeted by the killer because of her looks or appearance, which would be similar to one he possessed in his mind and was the reason for his mental anxiety.

The subject would be an intelligent person who is socially adept. He would not find conversation with another person difficult and would probably have been a professional person or possess certain skills in his employment. His objective would be to control each of his victims and obtain a sense of power and complete domination. He did not have to commit the crimes for any reason except self-gratification, and would have enjoyed what he had done. This is supported by the specific injuries inflicted upon his victims and the fact that he carried his knife with him to and from each murder scene.

In those cases where the victims were subjected to facial trauma, there could be two reasons for such actions. Firstly, the killer rejected the opportunity to look into the victim's face for a reason connected with his psychosis, or the victim's face reminded him of a traumatic experience from the past. The result was one of depersonalization.

There is little doubt that the man responsible for the murders was familiar geographically with the Whitechapel area. He was comfortable in the darkness of night, which he used as a cloak to escape detection, and rather than stalk his victims, having selected them, he prowled the streets looking for a likely subject. He would probably be of smart appearance because of the reduced risk of being challenged in such a poor area of London.

As far as age is concerned, the killer would most probably have been older than his victims. Because of the nature of the attacks it is unlikely that he was a young person. He would be between his late forties and mid-fifties.

On the night of the double murders, the killer would have committed the second crime out of anger, having not been able to fulfil his desires with the first victim.

The majority of serial killers operating in the United States of America, where such people are more common than in this country, move from an area in which they have been operating after a certain period of time. This would probably be the reason why after the fifth murder no others took place.

Thirteen

The Trial of Jack the Ripper

'To every subject in this land, no matter how powerful, I would use Thomas Fuller's words over 300 years ago: "Be you never so high, the law is above you." '

(Lord Denning MR in Gouriet v. Union of
Post Office Workers 1977)

In English law the burden of proof rests on the shoulders of the prosecution. A person's guilt has to be proven 'beyond all reasonable doubt' before a jury can convict. This basic principle of law has existed before and since the Victorian period. Nothing has changed during the past one hundred years. An adversarial system existed in 1888 and has remained the preferred system of justice in this country today. A person is tried for whatever crime he or she is alleged to have committed by a jury of their peers. The structure of a trial will include counsel for the prosecution, whose responsibility will be to place before the jury evidence which tends to prove a person's guilt. Counsel for the defence will try and rebut the prosecution evidence by presenting to the jury facts and opinions that will assist in proving a person's innocence. A trial judge will sit as referee to ensure that all of the legal procedures are adhered to by the parties involved, and then it is for the 12 men and women to consider the weight of evidence put before them and decide on the guilt or innocence of the accused person.

In 1888 it was the decision of the police as to whether or not a person was prosecuted for a crime. That procedure existed until a few years ago. Today, that decision is the responsibility of the Crown Prosecution Service, an organization that acts independently of the police. It is widely accepted, however, that because of the nature of the work undertaken, in many cases a close liaison exists between both the prosecutor and the police. The role of an investigating officer is to collect all the facts to a case and submit them to the CPS for a decision as to whether or not an accused person is arraigned before the courts.

For the crime of murder, which is the most serious in the Criminal Justice System, the powers of sentencing have changed during the past 40 years. When a person is found guilty of murder in this country, the trial judge has no alternative but to sentence the convicted person to life imprisonment. In 1888, the sentence was also mandatory: 'To be hanged by the neck until they were dead'. Such a punitive measure encouraged defence lawyers to represent their client with strength and vigour, to ensure that everything possible was done to provide the best defence for the accused.

This chapter will concentrate on the administrative and procedural issues that exist within the judicial system and structure today, although there is little difference between current practices and the way in which a trial was conducted in 1889.

On 2 April 1889, Andrea Chekensovsky was charged with the following offence:

'That you did on the ninth day of November 1888, during the reign of our Sovereign Lady Queen Victoria, murder one Mary

210

Jane Kelly in Whitechapel, London. <u>Contrary to the Common Law</u>.'

Abberline wanted to delay any further charges until he had consulted further with the Crown Prosecution Service.

On the morning following the charge, the Russian seaman appeared before the local Whitechapel magistrates, when an application for a remand in custody took place. The small Victorian court was packed with members of the public who wanted to catch a glimpse of the notorious Jack the Ripper. The press were also there in force, but seating was restricted on a first come, first served basis.

The court was a dark, oak-panelled room, with the dock situated in the centre facing the magistrates' bench. There was a hostile atmosphere, felt even by those who were merely observers. The Clerk of the Court, who was seated in front of three large high-backed chairs which would be occupied by the presiding magistrates, gazed around him, looking hard towards the people gathered. He wanted no breaches of decorum, and was prepared to jump on anyone likely to create a disturbance.

The walls of the dock were quite high, requiring people who were seated in the courtroom to look upwards to view those who would be standing inside. The only offer of comfort for a prisoner was one of three hard wooden stools placed in the dock for the use of the defendant and his escorting officers.

Chekensovsky sat in the smelly and damp windowless cell situated beneath the courts, waiting to be summoned up the winding stone steps which would lead him into the dock and the brightness of the courtroom. He couldn't see his hand in front of him because of the darkness. He thought of what he had told the interviewing officers, about feeling comfortable in the dark. This was a different kind of blackness, one which wasn't there to protect him, but to make him feel nervous and degraded. Against a background of keys jangling and the echoing of footsteps walking across the bare stone floors, he occasionally heard voices from outside in the corridors.

'That's him in there.'

'The Ripper?'

'Yeah.'

'God help him when he gets to the nick.'

Short bouts of laughter would accompany remarks about his future, which caused him to feel suicidal.

At the same time, Abberline was facing other difficulties. The Senior Investigating Officer had not intended to make an appearance at the preliminary hearing, but the lawyer representing the Crown Prosecution Service had asked for his attendance in case there were issues that required clarification. Now the inevitable had happened, and Abberline found himself subjected to a barrage of questions from a multitude of reporters who had painstakingly waited for his arrival since the early hours of that morning.

There was no news available for them as far as the police were concerned, because nothing could be said about the case now that a man had been charged. However, the media were persistent, and eventually Abberline had to summon the assistance of two burly uniformed officers who helped their senior officer make his way through the main hall of the building into the comparative safety of Court Number Six, in which the remand was to take place. There were streams of people standing in lines that started in the street outside the main entrance to the courtroom building and continued inside the premises up to the very door of the court.

A member of the Crown Prosecution Service welcomed Abberline. She was a small but fairly plump woman with long dark brown hair, who looked at the police officer with extremely sharp eyes. She asked a number of questions relevant to police objections to any application for bail, but explained that she felt it very unlikely that the defence would make such an application. Also present in court and slumped on the front bench was a defence lawyer. He looked directly towards Abberline, nodded and smiled, and then returned to the papers laid out before him. Abberline positioned himself near to the witness-box in case evidence of arrest or other proceedings was needed.

Following the entrance of the three magistrates, the Clerk of the Court stood up from his seat and called for order. There was silence and everyone, perhaps with the exception of the detective officers present, looked towards the dock. The sounds of loud, multiple footsteps could be heard climbing stairs from beneath the courtroom. Chekensovky's appearance was greeted by whispers that raced around the public gallery, which was situated at the back of the room. Everyone could see that the prisoner was manacled to two prison officers who stood at each side of him. The whispers stopped and the courtroom suddenly erupted into boos and hissing. A small, slightly built man who was sitting on a bench at the side of the dock immediately started to sketch Chekensovsky's face, obviously for the benefit of the early newspaper editions. Other members of the press were frustrated that they were not allowed to take photographs, but a number of reporters had already started talking into portable Dictaphone machines. The clerk shouted for order once again and banged his wooden anvil down hard, threatening to clear the court if any further disturbances took place. The Dictaphones disappeared and some resemblance of order was restored.

'Prisoner in the dock stand and face their worships,' requested the clerk.

Chekensovsky was already standing and facing the magistrates, and the clerk continued. 'Are you Andrea Chekensovsky?' There was a shout of 'Jack the Ripper' from the public gallery, but the clerk chose to ignore that particular jibe.

The answer from the dock was, 'Yes.'

'Do you reside at 23 Cavell Street, Whitechapel?'

'Yes.'

The clerk then read the charge out to the prisoner and told him to sit down. The Crown Prosecutor stood up and addressed the magistrates. 'As you are aware, Your Worships, the prisoner is charged with the most serious offence of murder. There are numerous enquiries yet to be completed by the police into other similar offences, and the application before you today is that the defendant be remanded in custody for an eight-day period. I understand from my learned friend that there is no application for bail.' She sat down immediately as the defence lawyer stood to his feet.

'No application, Your Worships.'

Both solicitors were now seated when the Chairman of the Bench, a grey-haired gentleman sporting both moustache and beard, whose face was more than familiar to those who regularly visited the courtrooms, ruled, 'Very well, case remanded as requested. There will be no bail.'

Chekensovsky signalled to his solicitor to see him later downstairs, and was ushered out of the dock back down the steps which he had earlier climbed. The courtroom was cleared in three minutes. People rushed out to tell friends and others about what had happened and to try and describe what the Ripper looked like, whilst the members of the press rushed to communicate the news to their different organizations.

Upon returning to Scotland Yard, Abberline immediately called a meeting of his Management Team and requested a full briefing for all officers and support staff later that afternoon. His message to his senior officers was short and clear. He thanked them for everything they had done so far, but reminded them that the job had not yet been completed and there was still a rocky road in front of them. The long laborious task of collating all available evidence and preparing a prosecutions file for the Crown Prosecutions Service was facing them. Each member of the Management Team was given new responsibilities. One officer was given the job of assisting the senior scientist with co-ordinating the forensic evidence. Another was to ensure that outstanding investigations were completed as soon as possible. Another senior detective was given the role of searching for and examining every item recorded on the Major Incident Room computer system, to list details for disclosure to the defence. It is the responsibility of the police to disclose all aspects of an investigation to the defence, with the exception of information that would not be in the public interest to disclose.

Three senior officers were assigned to file preparation duties, which entailed the compilation of all evidential material pertaining to each of the murders for the information of the Crown Prosecution Service. One of those officers was also given the additional responsibility of maintaining a daily liaison with the CPS lawyers, to ensure that all of their requirements and requests were dealt with.

Within a week of the first remand appearance, the following summary of evidence was presented to Abberline.

Summary of Evidence

The Nichols Murder

A total of 43 different characteristics found during the examination of the boot-print impression left at the scene of the murder matched perfectly with a right boot found in Chekensovsky's room at 23 Cavell Street. The forensic scientist who made the examinations and comparisons was prepared to give evidence of the fact that the boot made the impression.

Fibre samples taken from the woollen cloak recovered from the defendant's room contained the same dye as the fibres found on the victim's clothing.

There were blood samples taken from nine different sites on the same cloak that matched the blood group of the victim.

The Chapman Murder

The boot-print impression found near to the scene was more vague in appearance than that found near to where Nichols' body was discovered, but there were four positive characteristics that matched perfectly with the boot recovered from the defendant's room. The forensic scientist was prepared to say that the likelihood of the boot having made the impression was good.

Samples of a red-coloured substance were recovered from the same boot and were found to contain a manufactured red dye, candle wax and lead. This substance was identical to samples taken from the floor tiles situated in the enclosed passageway at 29 Hanbury Street, and was identified as a form of floor-polish.

The sample woollen fibres taken from Chekensovsky's cloak contained the same dye as the woollen fibres recovered at 29 Hanbury Street. There were no blood samples identical with the victim's found on the cloak.

The Stride Murder

There was no forensic evidence to link the defendant to the victim or scene.

The descriptions given by the witnesses Marshall, Brown and PC Smith were similar to that of the defendant, and arrangements were being made for identification parades to be held in the near future.

The Eddowes Murder

Handwriting samples could not be matched with the writing on the wall found in Goulston Street.

The results of DNA Analysis on the samples of blood recovered from the public wash-basin in Dorset Street were identical with the defendant's DNA Profile. Forensic scientists would say that the possibility of the blood not being the defendant's was 1 in 50,000 head of population.

Samples taken from three bloodstains found on the woollen cape and one bloodstain found on one pair of black trousers recovered from Chekensovsky's room matched with the victim's blood group.

The Kelly Murder

The DNA Analysis of semen found at the scene matched with Chekensovsky's DNA Profile. Forensic scientists would say that the chances of the semen not belonging to the defendant were 1 in 100,000 head of population.

The description given by the witness Hutchinson of the man seen with the victim prior to the murder was identical to Chekensovsky. Arrangements would have to be made for an identification parade to take place in the near future.

Other Evidential Points

The knife recovered from 23 Cavell Street had a dark brown wooden handle, 5 inches in length, and a blade, 8 inches in length and half an inch at its broadest part, which tapered to a point. One edge was sharp, the other blunt. Home Office pathologists who performed post mortems on all five murder victims will say that the knife could have caused the injuries sustained by each victim.

217

There were traces of human blood found on the knife which have been matched exactly with the blood of Mary Jane Kelly.

Five different sites examined on one double sheet of newspaper revealed the presence of human blood. All samples matched with the blood grouping of the victim Mary Jane Kelly.

Three different sites examined on one double sheet of newspaper revealed the presence of human blood. Attempts to group each sample have failed.

Thirty-eight daily newspapers recovered from 23 Cavell Street carry details of all of the Whitechapel murders.

There is sufficient evidence from the statements taken from witnesses and documents recovered to prove the following:

Chekensovsky was present in London at the time each murder was committed.

The defendant's feet were a size 8.

The defendant confessed to all five murders during interview.

The above details, together with statements and other evidential material, were forwarded for the information of the Crown Prosecution Service. Two weeks later arrangements were made for Detective Superintendent Abberline and Detective Chief Inspector Davey to meet with lawyers from that department, to discuss the future progress of the case.

In the meantime, Chekensovky's lawyers agreed for an identification parade to take place. The venue was at Bishopsgate Police Station, and the defendant was brought there by prison escort. The following witnesses were asked to attend and did so:

William Marshall, James Brown and PC William Smith, who had made statements to the Stride investigation team, and

218

George Hutchinson, who had described the man seen in the Kelly enquiries.

Each witness looked at the line of 12 men, all wearing felt hats and sporting dark moustaches, through a glass window from a corridor outside the Parade Room. PC Smith and James Brown positively identified Chekensovsky as the man they had seen with Elizabeth Stride just before she was murdered. George Hutchinson positively identified Chekensovsky as the man he had seen with Mary Jane Kelly just before she was murdered. William Marshall failed to identify the defendant. The case for the prosecution was now complete.

Abberline looked up at the dome which stood on top of the Old Bailey Central Criminal Court. He noticed the way in which it appeared to be reaching up towards the heavens, as though communicating with some higher authority. Although the centre of London was extremely busy on that particular morning, with people scurrying about, going from place to place, and the usual din of carriage wheels and horses' hoofs clattering along the cobbled streets, the air was fresh and the sky sunny and blue. Not really the kind of weather for sitting for half a day in some shaded room, discussing law and legal procedures.

Abberline and Davey made their way to the library on the first floor, where they were greeted by Mr Samuel Moffatt and Miss Greta Earnshaw from the Crown Prosecution Service. They were introduced by Moffatt to a third person present, Sir Charles Preece QC, who shook both officers by the hand and asked them to be seated in one of the heavily cushioned armchairs which Abberline found difficult not to sink into.

Moffatt opened the meeting by ordering coffee and biscuits. He then turned to Abberline.

'Superintendent, I received your file of evidence the other day and haven't really had a chance to study it in detail yet.

However, I have managed to run quickly through it, and have discussed my observations with Sir Charles here, who will be leading in the trial.'

Abberline looked sharply towards the older, silver-haired gentleman, Sir Charles Preece. 'Trial?' he asked, 'What trial? I thought that the evidence against Chekensovsky was overwhelming.'

The learned counsel nodded. 'It is, Mr Abberline, indeed it is. There is no better evidence than scientific facts, and that will, I am confident, secure a conviction.'

Abberline still looked somewhat puzzled. 'You said conviction, there are four more charges of murder which will be preferred before he is committed to take his trial. What about the confessional evidence he made to myself and Chief Superintendent Arnold?'

Sir Charles smiled. 'It is early days yet; let's not jump to any conclusions just yet. There is a long way to go, and I can only advise on the facts as they are put to me. Now all the evidence I have seen so far is of a positive nature, but we must look at how the defence will be thinking. At the end of the day, their client is facing the rope.'

Davey's remark, 'And so he should', was ignored, and Sir Charles continued, 'There is little doubt that the accused is responsible for the Whitechapel murders, but a conviction for murder isn't cut and dried. If we examine the circumstances of each death, it does appear obvious that they are not the work of an ordinary mentally stable man. Would you agree?'

Abberline nodded his head, 'Yes, I know the circumstances all too well, Sir Charles.'

'Then no doubt you will accept that the possibility of Chekensovsky being regarded as a person who is either insane or mentally deranged is a strong one?'

'Go on.'

'There are various degrees of mental instability, but as the law stands at the moment, only one dividing line between being found guilty of murder and sentenced to death, or being unfit to even plead to the charge by reason of insanity. Of course the defence have to prove their client's state of mind. It is not for us to do so, but that is only one avenue they may decide to go down. Of course, they would need medical evidence to support their claim, and we would have the opportunity to introduce our own.'

Abberline asked, 'What if medical evidence doesn't prove him to be insane, but supports my belief that this man is an evil being who murdered those women out of self-lust and enjoyment?'

'Then they may well examine the prosecution evidence and challenge the strongest points.'

'But you said yourself that the strongest evidence is scientific and there is plenty of that.'

Moffatt entered into the conversation. 'Let us firstly look at the items that were recovered from 23 Cavell Street and are evidentially connected with the scenes and victims of each offence. The defendant has never admitted owning any of those items, with the exception of the knife. Is there sufficient evidence to show that he had ownership of the cape, trousers and boots, the newspaper with the bloodstains and the trousers? He could say that they were already there present in the room when he moved in, on the day before his arrest.'

Abberline showed his concern. 'But the landlord in Cavell Street wouldn't agree with that.'

Moffatt continued, 'We are only pointing out to you the avenues open for the defendant if he wished to put up a defence. His confessions were quite explicit but lacked detail. He could say that he spoke as he did out of fear or whilst under some sort of coercion.'

The meeting was interrupted by a knock on the door, followed by a young woman in a black and white uniform carrying a tray of refreshments. After a table was laid and those present were invited to participate in the coffee and biscuits, Sir Charles Preece took up the conversation.

'There is a lot of strong evidence against Chekensovsky, but it is our duty to point out to you the possibility that we could still go to trial and that you and the other witnesses need to be prepared.'

The meeting then focused on individual statements, which were summarised by Miss Earnshaw. Numerous points and issues were raised by the lawyers and adequately answered by the police officers. Three hours passed rather quickly before the meeting was concluded. Sir Charles Preece stood up with a broad smile on his face and declared that the majority of cases were won in participation of what the defence were planning. His final words to Abberline were the most comforting heard by the senior detective that morning.

'If this accused man was to escape the hangman's noose, could you imagine the public hue and cry that would follow? The trial judge will be aware of that.' He gave Abberline a reassuring look and bade him farewell. The three lawyers walked briskly from the room, followed by the two police officers, Davey carrying a list of requirements identified during the meeting.

During the following months a number of meetings took place between police officers and lawyers. Abberline only attended when he was required, but the majority involved other members of his Management Team. The time soon arrived when the defence gave notice to the prosecution that their client had been medically examined by two eminent psychiatrists. They had both declared him insane and unfit to plead. The prosecution arranged for the defendant to be examined by two other eminent psychiatrists. They were both of the opinion that he was mentally unstable but not insane, and fit to take his trial.

Because of legal restrictions the media had little to report, but the residents of Whitechapel continued to monitor the proceedings. The Ripper's activities remained the most topical subject of conversation throughout the district, as life in the East End of London slowly returned to normal. Although the horrors of what had taken place during the previous autumn never really went away, public confidence was soon restored in the police, and other news items started to divert people's attention in other directions. The courtrooms, however, were still packed out for every remand and appearance the accused man made. Abberline dealt with two more murder investigations in London during the next six months. They were both fairly mundane compared with the atrocities he had dealt with in Whitechapel.

Extra police officers were marched into Court Number Five at the Old Bailey for the commencement of the trial of Andrea Chekensovky. They stood in a circle around the dock as the accused walked up the well-trodden steps to stand and face the Queen's judge, who sat with a shoulder-length wig and red robes covering most of the upper part of his body. Chekensovky looked drawn and had obviously lost weight since his first remand hearing. He looked up at the public gallery behind him and gazed into the faces of the people, most of whom had queued throughout the previous night to guarantee their seats. Some were laughing at him, while others showed their disgust. Beyond the circle of blue uniforms sat the barristers and Queen's Counsel. The wooden benches situated at each side of the dock were occupied by members of the press. The court was in silence, far different from his previous appearances in the local magistrates courts.

Abberline sat by a group of reporters, just to the left of the dock, and for a moment he and Chekensovky stared into each other's eyes. The prisoner gave that same staring look which he had maintained during their interview on the day of his arrest. A vacant look that showed no feeling, no remorse, no contempt, no guilt, no innocence, yet seemed to pierce Abberline like a lance being directed into his eyes. In return, Abberline looked slightly pensive.

'Prisoner in the dock...' As the clerk read out the formal charges on the indictment, Abberline's mind strayed back to the scene of the first murder, that of Mary Ann Nichols, who was found lying near the stable gates in Bucks Row with her abdomen torn open. He fought back the tears that were beginning to swell in his eyes, as he remembered the physical state in which the Ripper had left each of his victims. He looked again directly at Chekensovsky, who was still staring back at him, paying no attention to what the court clerk was saying. 'Yes, you bastard,' thought the senior detective, 'I've got you now; not long before you swing, you callous bastard.' Chekensovsky nodded towards him as though he had heard his thoughts and was agreeing.

Legal arguments took up the first two days of the trial, whilst counsel for the prosecution and defence debated with the trial judge various issues and made numerous legal and procedural points. Doctors for the defence gave evidence as to the accused's mental condition. The majority of expert opinions were rebutted by medical experts called to give evidence by the prosecution. After listening carefully and attentively to the various arguments, the judge ruled that the strength of the prosecution's evidence was sufficient to show that the accused was in fact fit to plead to the charges on the indictment and that the defence of insanity had not been proved.

Chekensovsky pleaded guilty to all of the murders, with the exception of that of Elizabeth Stride. Further legal arguments followed, and eventually Sir Charles Preece conceded that to continue with a trial on the Stride murder count would be futile. The point made by the defence, that it would be a waste of public money when the accused had already pleaded guilty to four other counts of murder, was accepted. The judge then ordered the papers relevant to the murder of Elizabeth Stride to 'lie on the file', which meant they would be filed away for any future reference which might be deemed necessary.

Abberline gave evidence on oath of the circumstances and background to each murder the accused had pleaded guilty to. He described in detail the horrific injuries each victim had been subjected to and the consequential impact the crimes had had on the Whitechapel community. The court sat in complete silence as the police officer spoke. This was the first occasion the full details of the Ripper's reign of terror had been made public, and people in the public gallery sat with mouths wide open as if in a state of shock, consuming every word delivered to the court. The descriptive narrative concerning the death of Mary Jane Kelly brought gasps from various parts of the court, and even the judge seemed to fidget on his chair when specific details were described. There was only one question the judge asked of Abberline:

'Officer, in all of your experience as a police officer, have you ever known such violence used against human beings as was the case in any one of these incidents?'

Abberline simply replied, 'No, My Lord, never.'

Roger Smythe, the Queen's Counsel for the defence, knew he was representing a lost cause and showed it in his mitigating pleas for mercy. At one stage the judge actually waved towards the learned counsel to finish quickly his final speech.

After what seemed to be an eternity of legal banter, the prisoner was told to stand and face the judge. The court official stood behind the red-robed figure and placed upon the judge's wig a square piece of satin black cloth. Sentence was passed on the ninth day of November 1889, a year to the day after Mary Jane Kelly had been murdered.

'Prisoner at the bar, you have pleaded guilty to four of the most heinous and brutal murders most foul ever to come before these courts. The murders of four women, albeit common prostitutes, women who had the right to live their lives as they wanted. You not only took those lives away but then participated in acts which go beyond the reasoning and understanding of mankind. Your deeds had a devastating effect on the law-abiding people of Whitechapel, and you only appear before these courts today as a result of the dedication and commitment of the police officers who were given the awesome task of bringing you here. There is only one sentence I am permitted by law to pass upon you, and that is that you are taken from here to a place of lawful execution and hanged by the neck until you are dead. And may God have mercy on your soul, which is more than your victims had.'

Chekensovsky's pale face turned away to leave the dock and again looked towards Abberline. The police officer looked back sternly. The prisoner smiled and winked, showing for the first time that he was human after all.

Fourteen

Conclusions

The person responsible for the Whitechapel murders was never caught. It is extremely unlikely that the killer's true identity will ever be known, and yet the series of crimes that took place during that autumn of 1888 still attracts criminologists and academic researchers like a magnet attracts metal filings. Jack the Ripper is known throughout the world and is as famous as Scotland Yard itself.

During the time of the Ripper murders, the structure of policing as we know it today was still relatively new. The Criminal Investigation Department based at Scotland Yard had only been in existence for approximately 20 years, although the Metropolitan Police Force was formed in 1827. The fact that policing has advanced enormously since 1888 cannot be in dispute. Whether or not current investigative and operational strengths would have been sufficient to have identified and apprehended the Whitechapel murderer in a previous age, remains open for debate. That is a decision for the reader to make, having gained some insight into the methods and workings of today's police service.

A number of senior officers involved in the Ripper enquiries did make public their thoughts and opinions. Doctor Robert Anderson, the assistant commissioner responsible for the CID who had overall command of the Whitechapel investigations, categorically stated that the police were aware of the identification of the culprit. Anderson retired from the police service in 1901 and six years later wrote in his book, *Criminals and Crime*:

> 'No amount of silly hysterics could alter the fact that these crimes were a cause of danger only to a particular section of a small and definite class of women, in a limited district of the East End; and that the inhabitants of the Metropolis generally were just as secure during the weeks the fiend was on the prowl, as they were before the mania seized him, or after he had been safely caged in an asylum.'

He refused to name the subject he referred to because of the possibility of libel action. If Anderson's statement was accurate, then a number of observations should be made. Considering the amount of public pressure the police were subjected to at the time, it is surprising that the media did not become aware of such facts. It can be assumed that Anderson's revelations would have been widely known in police circles, and newspaper reporters would have been told at some time during or after the investigations. If such inferences had been made in the knowledge that they were false, then the retired police officer must have had genuine reasons for making them. It could well be that, as a prominent senior police officer, he found it difficult to accept defeat in such a high-profile case and sought a way to blunt the criticism that resulted from the failure to bring the case to a successful conclusion.

Abberline appears to have been less ambitious in disclosing his personal beliefs. Severin Klosowski was a Polish Jew who came to this country in June 1887, after qualifying as a junior surgeon in that same year in Warsaw. He was employed as a hairdresser in the Whitechapel district until he emigrated to the United States of America in 1890. He returned to this country in 1891 and again took up employment as a hairdresser in the Tottenham area, using the name of George Chapman, which he partly adopted from a woman he lived with. He later became a publican and was convicted in 1903 of murdering three women whilst cohabiting with them between 1895 and 1901. He was hanged for his crimes.

According to the *Pall Mall Gazette*, Abberline became convinced that Klosowski, alias Chapman, was Jack the Ripper. The newspaper printed two interviews allegedly given to them by the senior detective. The journalist responsible for writing the articles stated that he had been given access to a letter written by Abberline to Sir Melville MacNaghten, assistant chief constable CID at Scotland Yard.

'I have been so struck with the remarkable coincidences in the two series of murders, that I have not been able to think of anything else for several days past; not in fact, since the Attorney General made his opening statement at the recent trial and traced the antecedents of Chapman before he came to this country in 1888. Since then the idea has taken full possession of me and everything fits in and dovetails so well that I cannot help feeling that this is the man we struggled so hard to capture fifteen years ago.'

Not exactly the words of a man who, because of his position, would surely have known the identity of the Ripper, if Robert Anderson's allegation that he was in an asylum is to be believed.

Abberline pointed to a number of factors that supported his suspicions:

1. Klosowski had arrived in London shortly before the first Ripper murders.

2. He left the country for the USA after Mary Jane Kelly had been murdered.

3. The murders stopped after Klosowski had departed.

4. It was widely accepted that the murders could have been committed by a person having 'anatomical knowledge' and the skills of a surgeon.

5. Klosowski resembled a number of descriptive points given to the police by witnesses during the investigations. He was short in height and wore a peaked cap. However, he would only have been 23 years of age at the time the murders were committed.

Abberline totally rejected Anderson's allegation that the Ripper had died in an asylum. Also the details of the letter supposedly sent to MacNaghten are contradictory to the claims made by Abberline's investigation team that their senior officer believed a Russian anarchist, Dr Alexander Pedachenko, alias Ostrog, was the Ripper. It is not beyond possibility that Abberline changed his views following the formal closure of the investigations in 1892, when his investigation team acknowledged his personal beliefs, and 1903, when Klosowski was hanged. The senior detective was presented by his team with a walking-stick which had the face of Abberline's suspect, Pedachenko, carved on it.

There is some further confusion, however, in that, Donald McCormick, in his book *The Identity of Jack the Ripper* cites Dr Dutton's *Chronicles of Crime* that Pedachenko was the double of Severin Klosowski. He was employed as a barber-surgeon in Westmoreland Road, Walworth, and also assisted a Walworth doctor at St Saviour's Infirmary, which was attended by three of the Ripper victims: Nichols, Chapman and Kelly. There is little doubt that both Klosowski and Pedachenko were separate individuals who knew each other and might well have exchanged names on occasions for whatever reasons they had. It does appear, however, from research previously completed into the Ripper murders, that Klosowski was Abberline's main suspect.

Sir Melville MacNaghten was of the opinion that the Ripper had committed suicide, shortly after the Mary Kelly murder. In *Days of My Years* he concluded:

'Although…the Whitechapel murderer, in all probability, put an end to himself soon after the Dorset Street affair in November 1888, certain facts, pointing to this conclusion, were not in possession of the police till some years after I became a detective officer. I do not think that there was anything of religious mania about the real Simon Pure, nor do I believe that he had ever been detained in an asylum, nor lived in lodgings. I incline to the belief that the individual who held up London in terror resided with his own people; that he absented himself from home at certain times, and that he committed suicide on or about the 10th of November 1888.'

MacNaghten was referring to a Doctor Montague John Druitt, who was a 41-year-old Oxford graduate. He was last seen alive on 3 December 1888, and his body was recovered from the River Thames on 31 December. Druitt left suicide notes and in one addressed to his brother he stated that, '…*it would be best for all concerned if I were to die*'. He had been a fairly successful barrister until he was dismissed from his employment just prior to his disappearance. There is little evidence that indicates any strong reason why Druitt should commit suicide, but according to MacNaghten he was allegedly sexually insane. If Druitt had been the Ripper and the reasons for his suicide were related to that fact, it is surprising that, having left notes which referred to his intended suicide, he did not bother to mention the fact that he had savagely murdered five women.

Although Dr Druitt was MacNaghten's principal suspect, the once head of CID named two others. Aaron Kosminski was a Polish Jew who came to England in 1882 and by the year 1890 was receiving treatment for insanity. MacNaghten described him as follows:

> *'Kosminski, a Polish Jew, and resident in Whitechapel. This man became insane owing to many years' indulgence in solitary vices. He had a great hatred of women, specially of the prostitute class, and had strong homicidal tendencies; he was removed to a lunatic asylum about March 1889. There were many circs connected with this man which made him a strong suspect.'*

MacNaghten's third suspect was thought to have been a Russian Pole by the name of Michael Ostrog. He was a 'confidence trickster' or 'fraudsman', but MacNaghten described him more as an insane maniac:

> *'Michael Ostrog, a mad Russian doctor and a convict and unquestionably a homicidal maniac. This man was said to have been habitually cruel to women, and for a long time was known to have carried about with him surgical knives and other instruments; his antecedents were of the very worst and his whereabouts at the time of the Whitechapel murders could never be satisfactorily accounted for.'*

One major feature identified from all of these differing views and suspicions is that they were observations made by senior police officers involved in one way or another with the Ripper investigations. In the absence of some level of consistency in the reports and material passed on by those officers, the existence of a conspiracy to prevent the true identity of the Ripper from being disclosed is difficult to accept. Such an idea has been suggested on many occasions in the past by various authors. The police service, like other large organizations, leaks information, in a similar way to how a colander allows water to run through it. That situation would have been the same one hundred years ago, and any attempt to conceal controversial and vital information such as Jack the Ripper's name and address, would have most certainly been impossible.

Although the atrocities of Whitechapel have remained undetected, they did not prevent the police in this country from obtaining a reputation for professionalism and success envied throughout the world. The achievements that earned such respect and credibility were due to men such as Fred Abberline and his colleagues, men who throughout their careers carried out their duties with a belief in justice and fairness, but did not have access to the investigative tools available today.

The complete catalogue of enquiries made into the series of murders lacks a motive. It can be argued that the real missing link, which was the failure to reveal or accept the killer's intentions behind each murder, was the fundamental reason for the failure to achieve the success that was so badly needed. Without a recognized motive, the investigation team would have been disadvantaged to such an extent that confusion and the lack of reliable intelligence must have been prominent. It must, however, be accepted that the amenities and resources available in 1888 were not sufficiently adequate to accurately identify the Ripper's motives.

The Psychological Profile leaves little room for doubting that sexual gratification was the main purpose for the carnage that took place. If that was the case, then there would have been the possibility of semen being left by the killer at one or more of the crime scenes. At the time of the investigations, such substances would have been disregarded.

233

If traces of semen had been recovered from a scene or a victim, then there would have existed a strong likelihood of a DNA Profile being created. This would have provided the Senior Investigating Officer not only with sufficient evidence to convict the Ripper, but a considerable amount of personal descriptive information about the offender, which would have been extremely useful in the search for him.

There was physical contact between the killer and his victims. The most likely sites for fibre retrieval would have been from the clothing of the murdered women. Again, the information that could have been obtained from subsequent analysis of any item belonging to the killer could have helped to progress the investigation further and supported a conviction at a later date.

There are a number of questions that will never be answered and will continue to baffle experts in the future. In the fairly confined area in which the murders were committed, one major mystery remains. How did the killer manage to travel from one street to another without being seen? The increases in police beat patrols and the deployment of vigilance committees on the streets must have made it difficult for the Ripper to stalk his domain, yet he did so repeatedly.

Following the murder of Mary Jane Kelly, there is no evidence of others being committed in the Whitechapel district. The two facts that should have been linked and considered seriously were the extreme violence used in that specific crime and it also being the final act of savagery committed by the Ripper, as far as we are aware. If it was accepted that Kelly's murder was the reason for the Ripper to have stopped his activities, then there are a number of logical reasons that become apparent. The theory that Kelly was the victim sought after from the very start of the murders could be a realistic one. The mental state of the Ripper could have triggered a guilty conscience which stopped him from

234

committing further murders, although such a theory is doubtful if the Psychological Profile is to be believed. If the killer had, by his own design, moved away from Whitechapel following the murder of Kelly, then could he have stopped himself from continuing his vile deeds elsewhere? Again, when examining his profile, it is extremely doubtful that was the case. If his lust for butchery was so strong, then, like a drug addict needing a fix to survive, he would have been forced to carry on murdering until he was eventually caught.

It is suggested that there are only two logical reasons for the Ripper to have stopped his murderous activities: either his own death or incarceration.

Comparisons have been made between the Victorian Ripper cases and other, similar high-profile investigations: the Yorkshire Ripper, who murdered prostitutes over a period of time in the north of England; the notorious serial child killers of the 1960s and 1970s and the mass murderers who in the last 30 years or so have been successfully brought to book and are currently serving out their life sentences. They were all apprehended following intensive police enquiries, and there is little doubt that with the levels of professionalism that exist in today's police service, Jack the Ripper, if he was alive today committing his heinous crimes, would have been put into the 'detected' category.

Unfortunately, the condemnation and disgust created by the Whitechapel murders could now be viewed with some degree of imaginative romanticism. The suffering of people who lived in the East End of London, not least of all the victims of the Ripper, has been long forgotten, but there is some comfort that should still be recognized. There will always be serial killers for the police to hunt and bring before the courts. There have been very few who have escaped justice in this country. The Whitechapel murderer was one of them. If he lived today, committing his repulsive and most foul crimes of murder, he would be caught and brought before the courts of justice, to be dealt with according to the law. No such person is free at present, and the police service is totally committed to using all in its power and capabilities to ensure that such a person never again escapes the wrath of the law. Police forces constantly rehearse operational contingency plans, in preparation and readiness for the time when the next Jack the Ripper walks the streets of this country again.

As referred to previously, hanging on a wall at the Police Staff College at Bramshill is a walking-stick in a presentation case. It was presented to Abberline by his Murder Investigation Team and carved on the handle is a man's face. Below the presentation case there is an inscription that reads as follows:

The Whitechapel Murders

The Whitechapel Murders in 1888, commonly known as the 'Jack the Ripper' Murders, took place in London between August 31st and November 9th.

The officer in charge of the investigation was Inspector (later Chief Inspector) Frederick G Abberline, and this stick appears to have been presented to him by his team of seven detectives at the conclusion of the enquiry.

Whilst the murderer was never identified, it is known that Inspector Abberline favoured the theory that the Ripper was a Dr Alexander Pedachenko or Ostrog, an alleged Russian anarchist living in the London area at the time, and the head of the stick may well be based on his features.

The stick was found amongst the possessions of Ex-Chief Inspector Hugh Pirnie (Dorset and Bournemouth) by his son, Commander Ian Pirnie, RM, and presented by him to the college. Chief Inspector Pirnie served on the Directing Staff from March, 1950, to December, 1953.

John Plimmer

Inside Track

Steve Blade: army deserter turned armed robber.

DI Jack Priestley: dedicated police officer and crime fighter.

Two men, once childhood friends, now on opposite sides of the law. Blade and Priestley are dramatically reunited in a police interview room after Blade's bungled armed robbery attempt. Brought up in the same neighbourhood, their lives were set on very different paths, seemingly never to cross.

But face to face once more, Priestley – suspicious and disillusioned by the festering corruption within the force – finds common ground with his former friend. The two form an unlikely alliance and embark on a deadly battle against the evil in their separate yet interwoven worlds.

A searingly authentic thriller of police corruption,
armed robbery and the drugs trade.

John Plimmer

Running with the Devil

Ex-con Steve Blade and maverick police officer DCI Jack Priestley: both successful in their chosen careers, both unorthodox in their methods.

Chance dictates that the vastly different worlds of these childhood friends will be drawn together once again. Although the friendship is marked by conflict, when they are assigned to work, Blade and Priestley call upon the trust and loyalty forged during their boyhood. In a daring and supremely hazardous undercover operation, Blade turns mole for the police and their darkly mysterious Secret Squirrels.

The partnership exposes not only the extreme violence of the professional criminal underworld, but also the corruption and treachery present at the very highest levels of the British Government and police force.

The gritty and hard-hitting sequel to *Inside Track*.

John Plimmer

In the Footsteps of Murder

Focusing on a number of high profile murder cases, John Plimmer takes the reader on an investigative and disturbing journey into the minds of notorious serial killers and the methods of police investigation used to catch them. Using his experience as senior investigating officer on over thirty murder inquiries, Plimmer is able to view cases including that of the Yorkshire Ripper and the House of Horrors from a unique vantage point. Using inside knowledge of the facts and of the people involved, he critiques both the professionalism and incompetence of the methodology used. He also examines the emotive aspect of the work, exploring the ability of officers to distance themselves from the emotional upheaval of cases that spark such intense media attention.

OTHER TITLES BY JOHN PLIMMER AVAILABLE DIRECT
FROM HOUSE OF STRATUS

Quantity		£	$(US)	€
FICTION				
☐	INSIDE TRACK	6.99	12.95	13.50
☐	RUNNING WITH THE DEVIL	6.99	12.95	13.50
NON-FICTION				
☐	IN THE FOOTSTEPS OF MURDER	8.99	13.95	15.00

ALL HOUSE OF STRATUS BOOKS ARE AVAILABLE FROM GOOD BOOKSHOPS OR DIRECT FROM THE PUBLISHER:

Internet: www.houseofstratus.com including synopses and features.

Email: sales@houseofstratus.com
info@houseofstratus.com
(please quote author, title and credit card details.)

Tel: Order Line
0800 169 1780 (UK)
International
+44 (0) 1845 527700 (UK)

Fax: +44 (0) 1845 527711 (UK)
(please quote author, title and credit card details.)

Send to: House of Stratus Sales Department
Thirsk Industrial Park
York Road, Thirsk
North Yorkshire, YO7 3BX
UK

PAYMENT

Please tick currency you wish to use:

☐ £ (Sterling)   ☐ $ (US)   ☐ € (Euros)

Allow for shipping costs charged per order plus an amount per book as set out in the tables below:

CURRENCY/DESTINATION

	£(Sterling)	$(US)	€(Euros)
Cost per order			
UK	1.50	2.25	2.50
Europe	3.00	4.50	5.00
North America	3.00	3.50	5.00
Rest of World	3.00	4.50	5.00
Additional cost per book			
UK	0.50	0.75	0.85
Europe	1.00	1.50	1.70
North America	1.00	1.00	1.70
Rest of World	1.50	2.25	3.00

PLEASE SEND CHEQUE OR INTERNATIONAL MONEY ORDER
payable to: HOUSE OF STRATUS LTD or card payment as indicated

STERLING EXAMPLE

Cost of book(s):. . . . . Example: 3 x books at £6.99 each: £20.97

Cost of order:. . . . . Example: £1.50 (Delivery to UK address)

Additional cost per book:. . . . . Example: 3 x £0.50: £1.50

Order total including shipping:. . . . . Example: £23.97

VISA, MASTERCARD, SWITCH, AMEX:

☐☐☐☐☐☐☐☐☐☐☐☐☐☐☐☐☐☐☐

Issue number (Switch only):

☐☐☐

Start Date: **Expiry Date:**

☐☐/☐☐   ☐☐/☐☐

Signature: _____

NAME: _____

ADDRESS: _____

COUNTRY: _____

ZIP/POSTCODE: _____

Please allow 28 days for delivery. Despatch normally within 48 hours.

Prices subject to change without notice.
Please tick box if you do not wish to receive any additional information. ☐

House of Stratus publishes many other titles in this genre; please check our website
(**www.houseofstratus.com**) for more details.